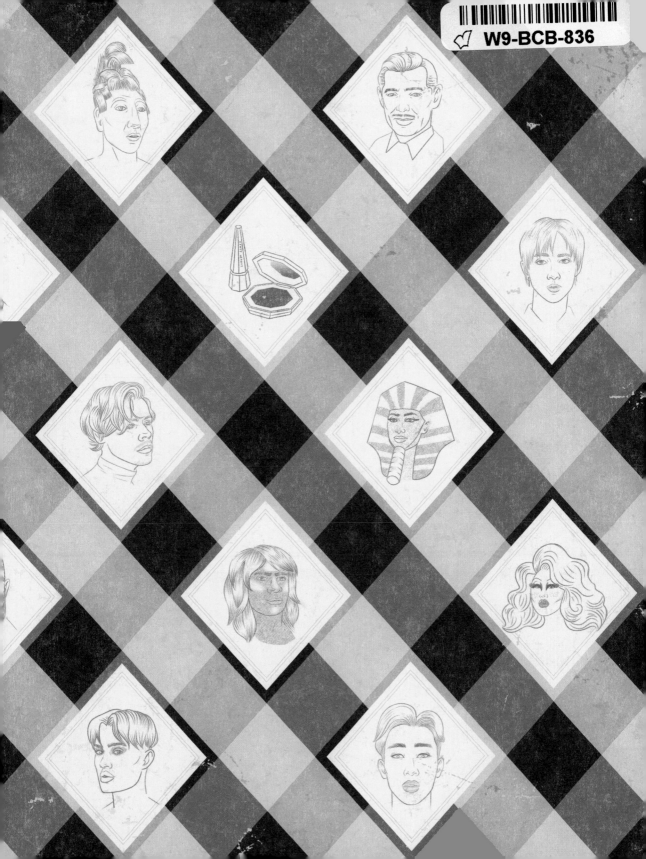

"The beauty industry is so important as it allows different demographics to feel seen and represented. But for far too long, the beauty industry has excluded men from the conversation. David transformed the beauty landscape by creating a safe space for guys to also participate not only in beauty, but find others like them. *Pretty Boys* does the same, showcasing men in all forms. When this book hits shelves, it will absolutely be revolutionary."

—CHARLOTTE CHO,
co-founder of Soko Glam and author of
The Little Book of Skincare

"*Pretty Boys* is not only important, it's culture-pushing. It also inspires anyone and everyone to embrace their authentic selves. We need a bold, beautiful, glittery beacon of hope more than ever and I know that that comes in the form of *Pretty Boys*."

—NICOLA FORMICHETTI,
artistic director and designer

"Before I became Patrick Starrr, I was like any other young boy trying to figure it all out. *Pretty Boys* is a beautiful collection of relatability that guides us through a similar emotion that many prominent people have felt throughout history. It proves that beauty has always been tied to all people no matter their backgrounds."

—PATRICK STARRR,
beauty guru and founder of ONE/SIZE

"It's time to learn your history, darling! David's storytelling and research bring to life the deep connections between masculinity and mascara! The idea of what a man is has changed throughout time, and keeps changing . . . so smear on some eyeshadow, draw on a lip, and bring out the 'Pretty Boy' inside!"

—SASHA VELOUR,
drag queen extraordinaire

"A visual journey worth your time. David's unique take on beauty is compelling and stunning, a must have."

—JONATHAN VAN NESS,
New York Times best-selling author of *Over The Top*
and host of *Queer Eye*

"In a political time that seems rather dark, it's encouraging to know we have a beacon of light. David has challenged the notions of masculinity since he started his mission and continues to do so with *Pretty Boys*. *Pretty Boys* is more important now more than ever and will certainly inspire future generations to push culture forward."

—JOE ZEE,
fashion editor and producer

"What I really love about beauty is that it makes me embrace the full power of Bretman Rock. But not everyone is comfortable with the power that is associated with feeling beautiful. This book proves that men and gender non-conforming people like myself have always used makeup and cosmetics as a way to elevate their look and spirit, giving themselves the power to change the world. Yes, pretty is powerful, and *Pretty Boys* has the receipts!"

—BRETMAN ROCK,
social media guru

PRETTY BOYS

LEGENDARY ICONS

WHO REDEFINED BEAUTY
and HOW TO GLOW UP, TOO

DAVID YI

ILLUSTRATED
BY
Paul Tuller

Library of Congress Cataloging-in-Publication Data is available
ISBN 978-0-358-41068-3

Book design by Raphael Geroni

Printed in China
SCP 10 9 8 7 6 5 4 3 2 1

사랑하는 부모님께 이승영과 신순진 바칩니다

Contents

*P*RETTY
POLITICAL

PRETTY FIERCE

Pretty
ICONOCLASTIC

....

INTRODUCTION

BEFORE MY FIRST DAY OF SEVENTH GRADE AT A BRAND-NEW middle school, when I should've been fussing over small details like the outfit I'd blow everyone away with or the lunch table I'd sit at, I was worried about something far more important: whether or not my new friends would call me gay. At an age when I was desperate to fit in, conforming was a means of survival. That meant hiding behind a broken facade of aggressive masculinity: the toughest kid in the schoolyard doesn't get picked on. So on that first day, I puffed out my chest, wore my jeans a little baggier, deepened my voice from soprano to tenor, and pretended that I was anything but who I actually was: a confused Korean American boy who was bewildered by—and afraid of—his identity.

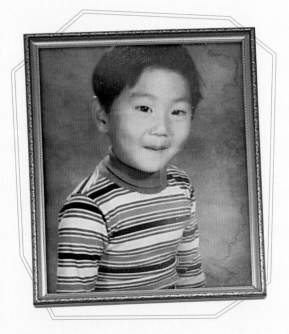

It didn't help that I had a Korean mother who was obsessed with protecting me from the sun. She'd slather my skin with sunscreen so thick, I ended up resembling a vampire by the time I got to school. And while beauty by way of skincare was normalized in my Korean household, it was a foreign concept to my American peers, who taunted me for it. To them, beauty was only for girls. Beauty was the ultimate act of feminine behavior. As a young boy, it meant you were *deviant*.

These dual identities pulled me in very different directions. I was taught that beauty isn't solely about aesthetics, that with every cream you layer, every drenching of your pores, you are engaging with a mindful practice of self-care and self-actualization. You're respecting and taking care of yourself. The West, on the other hand, equates skincare and beauty (or "grooming," to the men's beauty world) with weakness. Men are perceived as more "masculine" when they care less about their appearance and are encouraged to show their dominance through physical might and an aggressive personality.

Or at least, they *were*.

Fast-forward to today, when preconceived notions of "masculinity" are being challenged like no other time in recent history. In today's colorful world, people are discovering the freedom to express their identities in ways big and small. We're living in a day and age where exuberant stars from *RuPaul's Drag Race* are not only embraced, but celebrated as pop culture icons. This is an era in which men who paint their nails à la Frank Ocean or Harry Styles aren't automatically relegated to one orientation or the other. A time when the world's biggest boy band, BTS, is setting the new standard of male sex appeal with not only their talent, but their dewy complexions (and colorful hair!).

But did you know that eons before Chanel launched its men's beauty line, Boy de Chanel, cavemen had already created early forms of foundation and highlighter? In fact, thousands of years before Troye Sivan showed up on the red carpet with a multicolor mani, the ancient Babylonians were painting their nails in salons before battle. And centuries before K-pop boy bands and their makeup became international sensations, sixth-century Korean warriors known as *hwarang* used smoky eyes to channel a higher spiritual power while defending their kingdom from invaders.

So it's curious how history books emphasize the sheer brawn of men, particularly legendary historical figures, but fail to acknowledge their beauty—as if it somehow weakens or makes a man less-than. Centuries of heteronormative attitudes have minimized the close relationship men have always had with the ritual of beauty: to beat their foes, these men needed to beat their faces. To snatch some wigs, these leaders needed their own wigs snatched. For their legacies to grow, they needed to *glow*.

In this book, you'll read about how the radical act of beautifying for each of these pretty boy icons throughout history has always been more than the sum of their cosmetics and products—how beauty has acted as a channel for self-care and self-love. But of course, we'll cover both inner and outer beauty in this book: along the way, you'll pick up tips on makeup and skincare, and advice from the best makeup artists in the business—from Beyoncé's own Sir John to drag queen superstars like Kim Chi—in addition to meeting some inspiring contemporary pretty boys as well. They're all in here waiting for you.

Wherever you are on your journey—whether you're someone who cleanses their face with just water or subscribes to a ten-step Korean beauty regimen, already a beauty boy who celebrates yourself with a full beat and wig or simply a person curious about the history of masculinity and gender expression—this book is for you.

Before you get started, I hope you'll embrace this book on your own terms, and at your own pace. Think of the table of contents as a map, and choose your destination depending on what you need!

HISTORY BUFFS:

Travel to specific time periods to meet pretty boys of yore, uncover their surprising relationships with beauty, and experience the wide range of gender expression around the world and through the ages. (And in keeping with the spirit of the sheer diversity and fluidity of experiences within, don't be alarmed if you read one chapter and it's in a second-person perspective, then another reads like a love story, and yet another is like a mystery novel . . .)

BEAUTY ENTHUSIASTS:

Learn how to level up through tutorials from the best in the industry—get tips and tricks on everything from washing your face and taming your eyebrows to getting into your first drag look.

FOR THE COMMUNITY:

Get personal stories of self-actualization—from learning to love oneself to making beauty a brand—from *real* people throughout the world. Flip through the exclusive interviews with our pretty boys from around the world, or even start your journey at the end, and get inspired by ten modern-day pretty boys in the "What I Love About Me" section (page 240).

....

I've scoured the world and sifted through history books to discover examples and proof that men and masculine-identifying people did indeed beautify—but I realize this book doesn't represent the full scope of every human who's ever walked this earth before us. There are so many more equally important stories to include, so I hope this is just the beginning of this conversation about the gender-neutrality of beauty.

Writing and researching *Pretty Boys* has allowed me to finally come to peace with who I am. This has been such a healing process for me. Looking back, I know of one boy who struggled over the years to accept himself. In those lonely moments of confusion and self-loathing, he could have used a book like this to show him that he was perfect just the way he was. So to those of you out there questioning whether you can think of yourself as beautiful right now . . . yes, you absolutely can. You are, in fact, *stunning*. And I hope that the following pages will help you realize that your *pretty* has and will always be *pretty powerful*.

HERE'S to YOU, PRETTY BOY . . . MAY YOUR INNER and OUTER BEAUTY LIGHT the WAY.

Why Did Men Stop Wearing Makeup?

The hypermasculinization of man and how heteronormativity won out—until now.

AROUND 50,000 YEARS AGO, OUR COUSINS, NEANDERTHALS of all genders, painted their faces with foundation and highlighted their cheekbones with dazzling ground pyrite. In the centuries that followed, men utilized skincare and makeup as means of expression in tribes and cultures throughout the world. From pharaohs, kings, and warriors to everyday people, the practice of beautifying has held a wide range of purposes, from ritual to empowerment to survival. Yet fast-forward to our Western societies

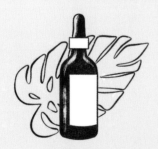

in the twenty-first century, where men wearing makeup has become a highly stigmatized practice, one that may attract disapproval from families, employers, and random nosy people on the street. How is it that beautifying has moved so far away from the concept of masculinity? For that, we must look back to the 1700s.

Until the mid-1700s, it was as common for men to express themselves through makeup and cosmetics as it was for women. Take the trendsetting pretty boys (and girls) of this century: the big-wigged French, lavishly dressed Italians, and red-lipped British. But by the end of the eighteenth century, culture had changed drastically. Of course, beauty was a vital part of cultures outside the Western hemispheres—this very book delves into many of them. But it was ultimately the Western models of stigmatizing beauty that dominated, due to colonization and a bid to view the world through a European lens.

In *Making Sex: Body and Gender from the Greeks to Freud,* author Thomas Lacquer argues that our contemporary gender binaries were created during the Enlightenment. Up until then, men and women were viewed as physically the same, which explains why it was acceptable for both sexes to partake in beautifying. But Lacquer makes a case that many Enlightenment thinkers from France to Great Britain pushed the idea that women were actually underdeveloped versions of men.

Historians call this period "The Great Male Renunciation," a moment in British history in which identity and its expectations became defined and separated by the gender binary. The name was coined in 1929 by Dr. John C. Flügel, an American psychologist and historian who noted that this was the era when men "abandoned their claim to be considered beautiful" and "henceforth aimed at being only useful."

And while women were being marginalized, men who refused to conform to more "serious" versions of masculinity were silenced, as open criticism in opposition to monarchs and the aristocracy also spread to associated frivolous practices, including beauty, that weren't essential to the common man. Though men from all backgrounds participated in grooming habits, it was really the upper class who were afforded the luxury to not only purchase beauty products, but seek out barbershops as a regular service.

Activities such as caring for clothing, cosmetics, or any type of self-expression were now considered feminine. Men's corseted clothing styles from Italy were replaced with three-piece suits and boxy silhouettes. Extravagant wigs were frowned upon and quickly went out of fashion. Modesty became de rigueur as Macaroni, the trendsetting "hipsters" of the eighteenth century, who once wore stark-white makeup, blush, and lipstick, were replaced by somber wet-blanket (or, in this case, makeup-wipe) Victorian-era socialites.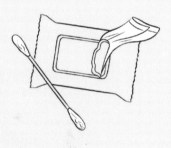

The Victorian era would systemically police all the fun out of expression—a situation only exacerbated by the 1800s obsession with colonization and war. With Europe racing to plant their flags on foreign soil, war not only propelled violence, but further spread Western, colonized definitions of hypermasculinity. By this time, brooding men like Beau Brummell gained respect and notoriety, redefining how dignified people were supposed to act, behave, and look. Beauty boys were deemed immoral, out of touch, and began to get erased from culture. A wave of anti-queer sentiment was ushered in, in which men who were interested in activities now coded as "feminine" were perceived as weaker beings.

By the late 1800s, male beauty and queerness were criminalized and deemed a "gross indecency" by the Criminal Law Amendment Act of 1885. In the new century, around 1924, a man named Thomas B. was sent to prison for three months for having a "lady's powder puff, powder and small mirror" on him. In court, prosecutors said that "the man who owned a powder puff was effeminate; the effeminate man possessed illicit sexual desires; such a man was . . . of the 'male importuning type.'" Later, William K., a hotel porter, was sentenced to nine months of hard labor and a whipping after authorities found "face powder, scented handkerchiefs, and two photographs of himself in woman's [*sic*] costume," and many others would be punished for similar "crimes" over the years.

America had also adopted and developed its own version of Britain's "Great Male Renunciation." After the American Revolution, leaders like Benjamin Franklin rejected fashionable items like the periwig, a popular wig in the 1670s with corkscrew curls parted in the middle. According to *Hope in a Jar: The Making of America's Beauty Culture* by Kathy Peiss, masculine American men were "expected to reject costly beauty preparations and other signs of aristocratic style." It was "unmanly" to have a desire for luxurious clothing, perfumes, or cosmetics. In 1840, members of Congress questioned President Martin Van Buren's masculinity by criticizing the cosmetics found on his desk. "Corinthian Oil of Cream and Concentrated Persian Essence no longer endorsed the gentleman of rank but intimated the emasculated dandy," Peiss writes.

The origins of American hypermasculinity were also fueled by politicians like America's ninth president, William Henry Harrison. He ran for office under the premise that Americans should embrace the "manly man"—a direct jab at Van Buren. He touted that he was born in a rugged log cabin and had "masculine" pastimes like drinking hard cider and being out in nature. When he was voted into the White House, the new president allegedly refused to wear a coat, despite record low temperatures—tough guys didn't need wimpy covering, he said. (He died from pneumonia a month later.)

At the same time, a misogynistic movement was sweeping the nation under the guise of facial hair, in response to the women's suffrage movement. Horace Bushnell, an influential pastor, had published a book called *Women's Suffrage: The Reform Against Nature,* in which

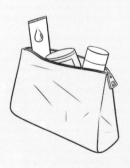

he detailed how women could never be equal to men, again because of their anatomy. "The man is taller and more muscular, has a larger brain, and a longer stride in his walk," he wrote. "In physical strength the man is greatly superior, and the base in his voice and the shag on his face, and the wing and sway of his shoulders, represent a personality in him that has some attribute of thunder. But there is no look of thunder in the woman. Her skin is too finely woven, too wonderfully delicate to be the rugged housing of thunder." Thus, big bushy beards, curled-up mustachios, extended sideburns, and more made a resurgence in the West.

At a time of political, social, and economic upheaval, facial hair was a symbolic reminder that men were still in control. Sprouting any facial fur in a variety of shapes and styles demonstrated dignity, virility, a demand for respect. "A woman trying to be in power was as ludicrous as a woman trying to grow a beard," was the defensive saying. Sure, a woman could vote, or protest in the streets—but could she sprout a thick mustache? Beards gained steam and continued to represent power into the new century, with presidents like Abraham Lincoln and his distinctive beard and William Howard Taft sporting a shaggy mustache in the early 1900s.

Ironically, in the twentieth century, this fueled a new "grooming" industry (calling it "men's beauty" was far too effeminate) to take care of men's beards. A growing number of barber shops and grooming businesses began popping up across the country, spaces where men would go to get a shave, have their hair cut, and . . . be away from women. On the other hand, revivals of Christian modesty led to women being stripped of beautifying rights—by the early 1900s, the only women who wore makeup were thought to be sex workers.

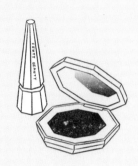

The world wars would reinforce and further entrench the divergent expectations around gender expression. As fathers, brothers, and husbands were drafted, leaving their newly vacant jobs needing replacements, the US government turned to women to fill these roles. These positions included manual laborers for the US Postal Service, drivers, factory workers, and more. Yet even as more women entered traditionally male fields, the cultural script flipped: women suddenly needed to be hyperfeminine, wear stockings at all times, paint their faces every day, and style their hair. New propaganda from cosmetics brands insisted that men needed inspiration while they were away fighting (hence the rise of the pinup girl) and when they came back home. "Beauty on Duty Has a Duty to Beauty," preached one ad that circulated in every newspaper. A 1941 article in *Vogue* reinforced this idea: "To look unattractive these days is downright morale-breaking and should be considered treason."

The biggest beauty campaigns to date debuted in the 1940s. Major brands like Tangee lipstick promoted the insidious idea of female fragility, and commodified femininity in relation to beauty: "Beauty—glory of woman [*sic*]. Liberty—glory of nations. Protect them both," one advertorial read. "Beauty must be served . . . on duty as well as off," stated another from 1944. Executives of brands like Elizabeth Arden went even further, creating an entire makeup kit for the US Marine Corps Women's Reserve, providing a lipstick shade that matched their uniforms. Helena Rubinstein debuted lip shades called "Fighting Red," "Commando," and "Regimental Red." The wars would create a boom in the cosmetics industry, but would lead to deep polarization: beauty products were feminine, while belligerent, soldierlike behavior was masculine.

The generational shift in understanding gender from the 1800s, reinforced by capitalism, would shape our contemporary view of identity into a restrictive binary with men as emotionless, macho heroes, and women as their beautified cheerleaders.

BUT TODAY, for THE FIRST TIME in CENTURIES, WE ARE WITNESSING a DEMOCRATIZATION of BEAUTY, RUNNING PARALLEL to OUR FIGHT for EQUITY and PARITY in ALL FORMS.

Beauty is no longer relegated to the ruling and moneyed classes, a class shift that we'll see as the book moves through time. Aided by YouTube, Instagram, TikTok, traditional media, and cosmetics brands themselves, we're undergoing a culture shift in which people of all identities are questioning dated gender roles, sloughing off the binary, and refusing to conform to engrained expectations. Collectively, we are examining and dismantling the past two hundred years of oppressive patriarchal propaganda and erasure of anyone who didn't fit in with "traditional masculinity," all in hopes of stepping into a freer, nongendered tomorrow.

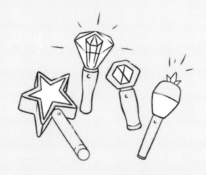

Now let's roll up our sleeves and rewrite history—the future depends on it.

Pretty

BEAUTY HAS BEEN A CONSTANT
SYMBOL OF POWER. IT HAS
ALSO ALWAYS BEEN A CONDUIT
FOR CHANGE.

Political

LET'S TAKE A LOOK AT THE MOST RENOWNED leaders and influencers in history—each of whom deliberately cultivated and used their outward aesthetics to amplify their sway over others. From Hatshepsut's beard to Louis XIV's wigs to the Black Panthers Afros, beauty has proven to be inherently political and political figures have used beauty—whether through makeup, hair, or facial ornamentation—to establish and demand new norms.

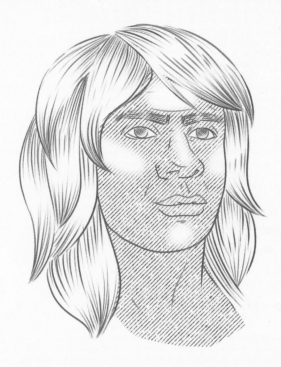

NEANDERTHAL

(5 0 , 0 0 0 B C E)

In the beginning, there was glitter.

EONS BEFORE KYLIE JENNER WAS LABELED A BILLIONAIRE beauty mogul (before getting stripped of the title), cavemen were grinding pyrite and mixing in different elements to daub onto their faces. Yep, the Neanderthal of 50,000 years ago invented foundation, color cosmetics, and glitter before modern humans—let alone Instagram—were even a *thing*. Which means we need to give a lot more credit to our long-ago, distant cousins. They weren't just simple-minded, low-browed creatures with inclinations to grunt and slam rocks together—they were actually highly emotionally intelligent beings who had the desire to enhance their aesthetics not only to showcase their beauty to others, but as a means of self-empowerment.

A 2010 mission led by archeologists from the University of Bristol in the UK analyzed pierced, hand-colored shells and mounds of pigment from two caves in Spain. At first, it seemed as if the findings were random mounds of colorful dirt and rocks. A scallop shell had remnants of orange, yellow, and red hues, which the team at first thought was evidence of paints that had been used for walls. But upon closer examination, the archeologists concluded that they were something extraordinary: the first known form of cosmetics. The yellow paints could have been used as foundation, while the red and orange powders may have been mixed to use as blush.

But the haul didn't stop there. The team discovered an amazing mixture of ground-up lepidocrocite (a lavender-colored rock), hematite (a strawberry-colored stone), pyrite (a rock with gold hues), and charcoal. Together, they created a stunning glitterlike substance. The effect, said lead professor João Zilhão, was a cleverly made cosmetic (similar to our present-day highlighters), both used over foundation. "Its preparation makes no sense unless it was used as a body cosmetic," Professor Zilhão told the *Guardian*. "When light should shine on you, you'd reflect." We now have a wide range of highlighters—from powder forms like FENTY Beauty's Killawatt Freestyle Highlighter to cream sticks like Glossier's Haloscope—but it's fascinating to imagine that tens of thousands of years ago, our distant relatives were also looking for that everywhere glow, whether on the forehead, cheekbones, clavicles, or, perhaps in their cases, to emphasize their striking brows.

Professor Zilhão also hypothesized a clear correlation between those who use makeup and cosmetics and emotionally and socially intelligent beings. To work to look your best and to flaunt your features—whether you choose to go with a natural, dewy face, or a full face of makeup—correlates with a greater capacity to think about one's social structures, whether to emphasize one's status or to blend in with the crowd. This trove of ancient highlighters, foundation, and blush provides a fascinating glimpse into the importance of makeup in our earliest communities. "Pretty" might very well be a natural extension of who we are at our core, so to our modern pretty boys: glow on!

Many millennia later, *Homo sapiens* still use highlighters, in the form of creams, powders, liquids, and more, to get a status-enhancing glimmer. "I think highlighters give off the sense of radiance, youthfulness and that fresh feeling," says Anthony Nguyen, celebrity makeup artist to the likes of Adele, Jessie J, Christina Aguilera, and Katy Perry. But highlighter is not always about achieving a glow, nor is it simply about dewiness, Nguyen says. "It could just be a completely matte color that's not shiny but used to bring out your features. . . . You can still look radiant by playing with light and darkness in your face with a matte finish."

In this highlighting tutorial, Nguyen breaks the process down, and shares the best tips to help you find your best light.

1. START WITH YOUR SKIN TYPE.

Not all skin is equal. Some have oily skin, while others have dry. Then there are people in the in-between with combination skin (see page 36 for more on skin types and How to Wash Your Face). Nguyen suggests powdery highlighter for oily skin, creamy for mature skin, liquid for dry skin, and a little mix of all three for combination skin. "There's so many different formulas—it's about figuring what's best for you."

2. THE SHADE OF IT ALL.

For highlighters, think brighter tones. After you've put on foundation and gotten your face painted in, add highlighters as a last step. "I think usually it has to be maybe three shades lighter or more," Nguyen says, "but it's just all about blending it in with the contours of your face and your main foundations, so it can't just be super, super bright." Nguyen suggests a champagne color for light to medium skin tones. For medium to deep skin, a peachy highlight or a deep bronze gives you a natural glow. Of course, not everyone is looking to have a subtle shine (this is highlighting, after all!)—the good news is that most highlighters are superpigmented, so pick the shade you prefer, and you will shine like the gods.

3. TOOLS OF THE TRADE.

When it comes to highlighters, find the tools you need. Sometimes, all you need are your fingers. "When it comes to cream highlights, for instance, I personally love using my hands because your fingers can really help melt the product into the skin," Nguyen says. "Or if I'm using highlights that are matte and cream, then I like to use a sponge such as a Beautyblender or just a regular square sponge. If it comes to using powder highlights, then I prefer using a fluffy dense brush, and when you have a brush that's a bit more dense, it increases the intensity of the highlight, versus if it's just a brush that's a bit more sparse. It's gonna give you a bit more of a natural highlight."

4. MAP IT OUT.

Use your features to help imagine a grid to lay out where you want to highlight. The easiest way to see where your face is naturally highlighted is to put a light above your face and shine it downward, exposing the areas that are light and dark. Some may have more pronounced cheekbones than others. "It's about finding the high planes of your face," Nguyen says. Popular highlighting places: "Cheekbones, the bridge of the nose, above the brow bone, or right at the center of your eye where the tear duct is, top of the forehead, or the center of the chin." As a bonus: ears! "I like to include the ear as well and the neck so that everything looks even." Swipe on the tops of your ears and the sides of your neck—wherever the light hits.

5. YES, HIGHLIGHTERS CAN LOOK NATURAL.

For some, highlighting might seem too intense for a daily look. But to create highlights that are even more subtle than the above techniques, simply grab a foundation or concealer a few shades lighter than your own complexion and paint it onto the high planes of your face. Then pat loose powders in on top in a process called "baking" (aka locking in any product), and voilà—you've got a brighter yet still natural look that'll draw the eyes of those around you.

PUT A LIGHT ABOVE YOUR FACE AND SHINE IT DOWNWARD,
EXPOSING THE AREAS THAT ARE LIGHT AND DARK.

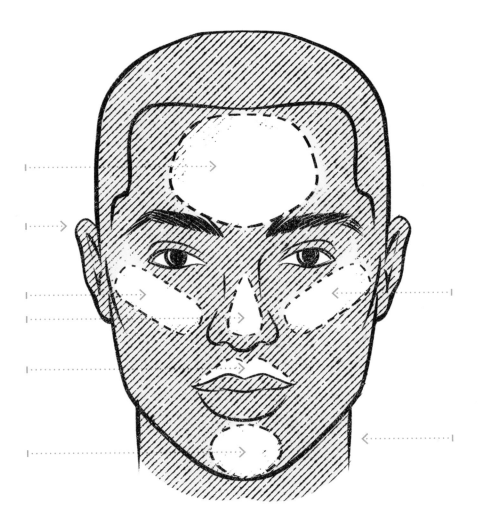

IT'S ABOUT FINDING THE HIGH PLANES OF YOUR FACE.

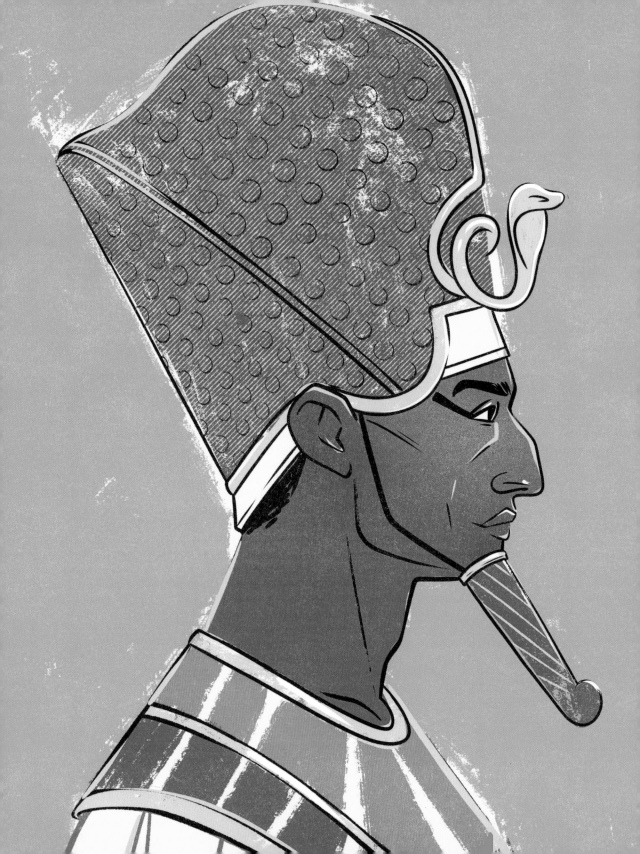

RAMSES THE GREAT

(1 3 0 3 - 1 2 1 3 B C E)

A ruler's extensive and blessed morning regimen, explained.

IT'S ONLY DAWN AND ALREADY DOZENS OF ASSISTANTS ARE working furiously around the clock. In one corner is a wig station where stylists are gliding brushes through silky strands of hair. In another, manicurists have set up basins full of fragrant water mixed with drops of exotic oils. Makeup artists line tables with beautiful eyeshadow pigments in scintillating emerald, gold, and black, making room for the aestheticians to organize rich creams, moisturizers, and exfoliators, all sourced from the most expensive ingredients.

If you're thinking this is the setup for a royal wedding, or perhaps a *Vogue* cover shoot for Beyoncé, you probably wouldn't be wrong. But this would actually be just another morning for an Egyptian ruler like Ramses II—better known as Ramses the Great—who was accustomed to being primped and pampered for hours on end before his day even began. And this wasn't for #selfcare reasons alone—for the ancient Egyptians, the better you smelled, the more attractive you looked, and the glowier your complexion, the more favorable you'd be in the eyes of the gods.

The ancient Egyptians lived by a strict set of hygiene rules that were codified in religious texts like the *Book of the Dead*. According to it, one couldn't even open their mouth to speak in the day unless they were "clean, dressed in fresh clothes, shod in white sandals, painted with eye-paint, anointed with the finest oil of myrrh." Any pressing matter, from defense strategies for protecting the kingdom from neighboring rivals like the Hittites to architectural decisions, would have to wait until one looked—and smelled—one's best. And so, every morning before sunrise, Ramses the Great would open his eyelids to find dozens of officials, servants, assistants, and slaves waiting to guide him through his elaborate beauty routine—a collective of people and products that may be the original beauty industry.

Led by a person literally named the "Chief of the Scented Oils and Pastes for Rubbing His Majesty's Body," one of the most important people in Ramses's palace, the staff would start by dunking his body into a warm bath, sometimes filled with milk. The team would scrub every square inch using soaps made with animal and vegetable oils mixed alkaline salts found in the Dead Sea, a natural antibacterial. While he soaked in the water, they'd mix milk and honey to create face masks, slathering them across the pharaoh's bronzed face for a thorough exfoliating and moisturizing treatment. If they had time, they'd remove hair from his body through a process called sugaring, in which the hair is removed with a mixture of sugar and honey. Before he was dressed, he would be doused in a potpourri of perfumes.

> One of the best known and favorite perfumes of royals was kyphi, a rare and luxurious fragrance composed of mastic, pine resin, cinnamon, frankincense, myrrh, mint, and other aromatics. The scent was sweet, spicy, and long-lasting. Kyphi was so expensive, it's said that it was used sparingly for mortals, relegated mostly to temples where it would be burned for the gods.

Afterward, manicurists would be summoned to trim his finger- and toenails with a small file and knife. The position was of such importance and high esteem that many manicurists would later include their job title front and center on their tombs. To touch the hands of a pharaoh, whom they viewed as godly, was the greatest of honors. So was clipping his toenails.

With Egypt's scorching climate (with heat going up to 122°F), it was essential that creams, moisturizers, and masks were layered on the pharaoh's face multiple times throughout the day to keep his skin supple.

> One such recipe was an antiaging cream made of honey, lotus flowers, and plant oils, including papyrus. The cream was also a multitasker: effective at fading scars, acting as a sunscreen, and a natural insect repellent.

After Pharaoh's face was softened and radiant, makeup artists would be summoned to line his eyes with kohl. Eyeliner was the most important step, according to Egyptologist Helen Strudwick, who notes that in ancient Egyptian culture, the eyes held great power. To accentuate the eyes, they were outlined with green or black paint, elongating their shape and size. Sporting the sparkliest, highest-quality eyeliner signified royalty and power—the ingredients in eyeliner were accessible only to the higher classes.

Ancient eyeliner was composed of pigments in green malachite and black kohl, made from grinding galena, a natural form of lead, with oil or fat, which created a creamy substance that would allow the product to last all day. Sometimes other luxurious ingredients were added for a glossy effect, such as ground pearls, rubies, emeralds, silver, gold, and coral, in addition to medicinal herbs like neem, saffron, and fennel. The liner would be painted on by hand or with a brush or small stick in a daily process, satisfying both aesthetic desires and religious obligations.

But as extravagant as eyeliner was, it also symbolized that the wearer had the protection of the gods Horus and Ra, who would ward off illness and evil." And wearing kohl eyeliner had its practical purposes as well. Before the advent of Ray-Bans, Egyptians found that rimming their eyes with a coat of eyeliner reduced the sun's glare, trapped dust and dirt and kept it from entering the eye, acted as an antibacterial agent, repelled insects, and provided cooling relief.

As the final step before Ramses II headed out the door, his stylists picked out the perfect wig to plop onto his shaven head. Wig selection was important in accordance to the tasks ahead in the day, and Ramses, like all pharaohs, had multiples ready for specific events like family gatherings, festivals, or war. Different wigs—commonly made of human hair, though horsehair wigs would later be introduced as a fashion trend—were adorned with gems, braided with jewelry, and cut to specific lengths. Wigs also prevented lice as they were worn over bald scalps, making it easier to maintain hygiene, and provided respite from heat. The ancient Egyptians even had beard wigs—gold plated, knotted, and worn hooked behind the ears—which were used more for religious ceremonies.

With his morning rituals complete, his skin moist and face dewy, Ramses was *finally* ready for his duties. He would begin the early afternoon with a first stop at the many temples where he'd pay homage to the gods and pray for their favor. Once he'd paid his respects, he'd head off to accomplish history-making feats: signing the first recorded peace treaty; expanding Egypt's territories and influence; commissioning some of the most breathtaking architecture in all of world history; and fathering two hundred children. Whew, he was booked and busy, but never too occupied for a facial. Ramses II's beauty rituals must have made him radiant indeed, to have received *all* those favors during his sixty-seven-year reign. There were eleven rulers named Ramses in Egyptian history, but only one was godly enough to bear the title "the Great."

If eyes are the windows to the soul, then eyeliner is the fuel that sets the house on fire.

Okay, not literally—we don't want anyone setting themselves on fire at the expense of this metaphor. But it's undeniable that eyeliner brings heat to any wearer's overall look. Since ancient Egypt, kohl has been used to outline the eyes, often smudged for a bold, smoldering effect. Fast-forward to the modern day, and kohl is no longer as popular as it once was, replaced instead by pencils and liquid eyeliners. But the intention remains the same!

Just ask celebrity makeup artist Jessica Ortiz, whose clients include actors Rami Malek and Darren Criss. Both are no strangers to eyeliner: the former used it throughout filming *Bohemian Rhapsody,* while the latter wore electric-blue eyeliner as part of his dazzling 2019 Met Gala look. Here eyeliner expert Ortiz walks you through everything you need to know to line your eyes like an Egyptian god (or Rami Malek, for that matter!).

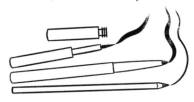

1. KNOW THY TOOLS.

Are you a pencil, gel, or liquid type of person? Identifying which tool works best for you is the first step toward lining your eyes. "Kohl pencils are easiest for beginners and can be smoked out to give a more grunge look, one that doesn't have to be so perfect," says Jessica. "Gels glide on easily and are a great next step once you have mastered the pencil." But they're not for the faint of hand: "They set quickly, so work fast!" As for liquid? That's for when you've mastered the first two: "Liquid eyeliners are more permanent and precise, and give you those perfect, deep, dark lines," says Jessica.

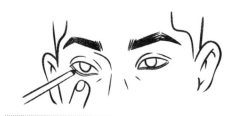

2. PRACTICE THE MOTION.

Whichever tool you end up using, applying it isn't going to feel natural at first. And everyone's different: "Some people's eyes immediately water, while others want to immediately clamp their eyes shut," Jessica says. "It's a natural reaction, so don't worry." When it comes to definition, you'll usually want to fill in the waterline—the flesh-toned area under and above the lids— as well as you can with a waterproof pencil. The waterline can be super sensitive, so Jessica suggests slowly allowing your eye's reflexes to get used to the feeling. "The more you try it, the less it'll feel weird."

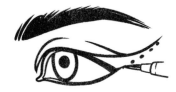

3. DOT IT AND DASH IT.

To line the actual eyelids, "Start by using a light touch, feathering the pencil at a slight angle gently. You'll soon be able to do a line in one swoop in no time," she says. For liquid eyeliner, use dots on your upper lid and then connect them with a line. If it doesn't look symmetrical or if you've messed up, don't sweat. Simply dip a Q-tip in micellar water and use it as an eraser. And if you're still not getting the lines perfect the first few times, don't fret. As Jessica says, "Not having perfect eyeliner on the first try happens to the best of us—it's all about doing it again and again until it's just right."

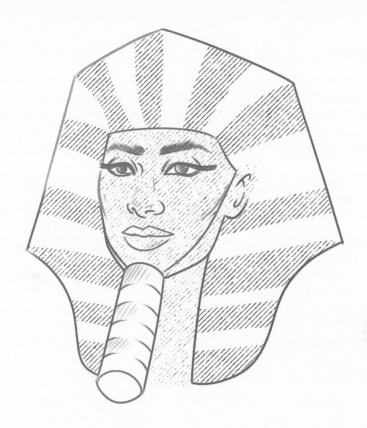

HATSHEPSUT

(1 4 7 9 – 1 4 5 8 B C E)

A ruler, their dual image, beard, and erasure.

IT LOOKED LIKE A BRUTAL MURDER SCENE: EYES GOUGED, BODIES decapitated, names scratched out.

The year is 1927, and in front of Egyptologist Herbert Eustis Winlock, then head of the Metropolitan Museum of Art, lay shards of broken granite and limestone. They're remnants within the tomb of a pharaoh named Hatshepsut. From the rubble, it's hard to imagine these broken pieces as whole, grand, proud statues.

As Winlock is excavating, he's unnerved. He and his team are aware of what this type of violation means, especially in ancient times. Egyptians viewed their pharaohs as gods. For anyone to have defamed the depiction of a royal—whether a painting or a statue—wasn't only malicious, but sacrilegious. Ancient Egyptians believed that the spirit would first travel through the underworld and be subjected to various tests and assessments of worthiness before finally reaching the afterlife. This, of course, only if their earthly effigies remained intact.

Who could have despised the pharaoh so much as to have attempted to erase their image from history—and with it, their spirit from thriving in the afterlife? Soon, Winlock would unlock the secrets in front of him. He just had to piece the mystery together first.

....

ALL HATSHEPSUT WANTED WAS A BEARD.

Beards signified royalty and power. Beards were signs of godliness.

But beards were only for men.

While her father ruled over Egypt, she observed him closely, taking notes on how he carried himself, his many decisions, his diplomacy, the respect he commanded. While she desired nothing more than to follow in his footsteps, her mother would tell her that the throne was no place for a girl.

The only child of Thutmose I and his chief wife, Ahmose, Hatshepsut was expected to be like her mother: beautiful, submissive, possessing all the virtues of a prudent wife. To young Hatshepsut, this was infuriating. A woman couldn't ask for the moon, but a man could have the universe.

Hatshepsut was married to her younger half-brother, Thutmose II, and after the death of their father, he became pharaoh. But Hatshepsut, though she was queen, soon found herself eclipsed by his secondary wife, Iset, and, even worse, by Iset's newly birthed son, Thutmose III. While they were promoted to becoming the new royal family, Hatshepsut, with her daughter Neferure (meaning "Beauty of Ra"), were moved to a lesser chamber. As Iset celebrated her new future as queen of the empire, Hatshepsut burned with envy, not of Iset, but of the infant prince.

When Thutmose II died a few years later, the empire mourned. Egypt desperately needed a stable ruler after two deaths in such close succession. But Thutmose III was a mere toddler. Regardless, bathed in myrrh, cloaked in royal blue, dripping with gold, the successor, wrapped in Iset's arms, was walked toward the throne for his anointment by the gods. But the throne was occupied.

In front of them was none other than Hatshepsut, sporting the sacred *khepresh*—the royal headdress with a golden cobra hooked to its front, its eyes glinting ruby red—along with a masculine leather kilt tied to her waist. Around her chin she had wrapped a false beard, braided from goat's hair, long and skinny to resemble that of Osiris, god of the afterlife. It was the ultimate sign of authority.

> *Egyptians were meticulous groomers and would shave their bodies from head to toe. A wig would cover a pharaoh's cranium. Pharaohs were living, breathing, earthly representations of their gods and they'd go to every length to resemble them. Beard wigs were sacred and symbolized ultimate authority. They came in two distinctive styles: The first was made of goat hair, either woven in a horizontal pattern or tightly braided to a long, thin point. These were strapped around the neck and pasted onto the chin to keep them in place. Sometimes the beards were held in place with cords that could be tied behind the head, then hidden with a wig. The second type was made of pure bronze or gold, with braided detailing. It would be tied to the khepresh so that it dangled from the royal headpiece.*

Up until that point, Hatshepsut had been depicted as female in the portrayals of her winding curves, the softness in her posture, in art. But now, wearing the false beard perhaps validated how Hatshepsut had felt all along: not fully woman, not entirely man, instead somewhere in between.

In the following years, descriptions of the pharaoh ranged from using "she/her" pronouns—"She Is First Among Noble Women," "Daughter of Re" (a feminine word ending)—to neutral—"His Majesty, Herself"—to simply "His Majesty." As such, from here on out, we will use they/them pronouns for the ruler. Monuments were erected that showcased the new pharaoh with chiseled muscles and a masculine posture. Hatshepsut's face was sculpted into a sphinx, a hybrid creature that the Egyptians viewed as male. Hatshepsut was a commanding pharaoh, commissioning a profusion of art and architecture, reopening trade routes with foreign countries, strengthening the royal army, and expanding the kingdom.

Yet Thutmose III would be waiting in the wings, as Hatshepsut once had. As a young adult, Thutmose III felt he deserved his rightful authority. But as he asked to be recognized, the royal courts denied his request to be the sole ruler, when they already had such a mighty pharaoh. To appease the petulant young man, Hatshepsut gave him distractions—lofty roles like leading the Egyptian army, and foreign missions far and wide.

As time passed and Hatshepsut became aware that their time as ruler was ending, it became imperative that they be remembered and memorialized alongside past pharaohs. For years before their death, Hatshepsut oversaw the building of a new burial structure alongside their father's. This would all but guarantee that their legacy and history would never be questioned, they thought.

When Hatshepsut died, all their people came to their tomb to pay their respects. But Thutmose III refused to attend. On the day of their long-awaited coronation, in a monsoon of rage, Thutmose III ordered that all monuments, portrayals, and paintings of Hatshepsut be vandalized. Strike out their name, remove their eyes, he directed. "Ensure that no one will ever remember Hatshepsut ever again!"

....

AND SO THE SINGULAR HATSHEPSUT WAS FORGOTTEN.

Until, standing amid the dust and rubble, Winlock came upon a single surviving inscription on one of Hatshepsut's obelisks. It was as if the late pharaoh spoke to him from the afterlife: "Now my heart turns this way and that, as I think what the people will say—those who shall see my monuments in years to come, and who shall speak of what I have done."

Taking the severed pieces, he and his team carefully pieced them back together, so that once again, we have proof of this genderfluid ruler and their accomplishments, never to be erased from history again.

"Now my heart turns this way and that, as I think what the people will say—those who shall see my monuments in years to come, and who shall speak of what I have done."

—HATSHEPSUT

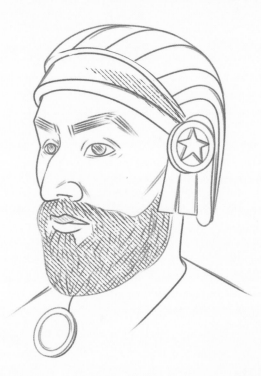

CYRUS THE GREAT

(6 0 0 - 5 3 0 B C E)

The Beauty King.

IT'S BEEN A DEVASTATING WEEK.

Your country has been defeated by your greatest enemy, the Persian Empire, whose king, you've heard, is as ruthless as he is dangerous. You recall your own father once warning you about this man, whom people call "Cyrus the Great." As one of the last surviving members of the court, you expect to go the same way, but you promise yourself to die with honor.

A voice interrupts your thoughts.

"Stand attention!" the Persian guard yells, his voice bellowing into the crowd. "Bow down to your new king."

In the distance, you make out a tall, regal figure on the horizon. You wipe your eyes to get a better glimpse of the mirage, draped in a fine, colorful fringed robe, his arms bedecked with golden bracelets that scintillate in the daylight.

You've heard so much about him, the founder of the Achaemenid Empire, the most powerful in the world. Under his leadership, his armies have conquered nations ranging from Western and Central Asia to the lands surrounding the Mediterranean Sea to the Indus River, where you're from. He has created the Persian Empire.

As you study the great leader in front of you, you're bewildered. This man isn't the brutish goliath you'd been taught to imagine.

His olive skin glows under the sun's rays. Moisture drips from his brow. His glossy lids smolder with dark kohl that resembles smoke, rising from the outer corners of his squinting eyes—he glances at you, and you feel flushed, as if wine has touched your lips. You can't help but stare at his grand hooked nose and his thick, curly facial hair, perfectly moisturized with what you're sure is expensive oil. His chiseled cheeks are dabbed with a deep rouge balm, blended into sun-kissed radiance. As he walks past you, a strong, decadent scent wafts into your nostrils, intoxicating your senses. You identify the fragrance: a potpourri of musk, myrrh, saffron, camphor, and other sweet-smelling plants.

King Cyrus is extraordinary—a true stunner.

In the upcoming weeks, King Cyrus invites you to join his royal counsel. You know your people best, he says. It'd be an asset for you to continue governing them. And so you wake up earlier than the sun to be taken to a salon. This is your initiation into the Persian Empire.

The salon has shelves full of colored glass jars in every hue. You're assigned your own personal makeup artist who awaits you, bottles of cosmetics in hand, a lush towel hanging over their arm. You melt into your seat and shut your eyes as the makeup artist takes kohl and pencils in your eyelids, blending them out onto your lids. Kohl, you're told, is important, as it makes your eyes "more lustrous than they are." Rouge is blended onto your cheeks to give you a flush of color.

As you'll learn, King Cyrus expects excellence from his employees, in all aspects. Beauty is no exception. The purpose of glamour is "to excel his subjects but also cast a sort of spell on them." You're to be better than those you serve so that they can look to you for hope—to be beautiful, to inspire admiration and awe, is a duty.

The dress code is Median, a traditional Persian costume of cotton, draped over you from head to toe. While elegant, it also has a practical purpose: it's flattering, concealing any physical insecurities you may have, while lending the illusion that you're taller than you really are.

You're told you can even use insoles in your shoes to elevate your stature further, if need be.

Your hair is plied with henna for shine, and dyed jet black with a dark mixture of indigo, oak apple, and walnut. Afterward, your hair is curled, softened with oils, and soaked in perfume so your locks "look better than nature made it."

As the makeup artist will explain, hair signifies a person's state of health. It reflects the strength, virility, and overall condition of one's body. You get a flashback to when you first beheld the king, and you can't argue that first impressions are indeed important.

An hour passes, and your look is complete. You glance at your reflection, and your mouth gapes open—you can't believe the glamorous person standing before you. A beautician will tell you this later, but you begin walking with a heavier step, your head held up higher, your chest puffed out with pride. As you walk into the king's chambers, he scrutinizes your new look, smiles, and nods. You're ready.

There are decades of prosperity under the Persian Empire. So much so that you now identify as Persian—much to even your own surprise.

When King Cyrus eventually dies, defeated in battle, you, along with millions of others, mourn with grief. "He honored his subjects and cared for them as if they were his own children and they, on their part, revered Cyrus as a father," the Greek author Xenophon will write later in a series-length biography of your king. You're relieved that his story will be memorialized. He did, after all, change your life for the better.

As one historian noted, "A man did not become king because he was handsome, it was because of his position as king that he was automatically designated as handsome." According to multiple sources, however, including the Cyrus Cylinder, a set of cylindrical clay tablets that retell his conquests, Cyrus the Great looked and acted the part of a perfect king. Various accounts, from the Greek Cyropaedia by Xenophon to the Old Testament, write fondly about his beauty, and recount how he was the first conqueror on record to support human rights. Though it feels strange now to see this type of adoration for a conqueror, Cyrus the Great would inspire generations to come, including the likes of Alexander the Great and Thomas Jefferson, both of whom perceived the Persian king as a superb example of leadership.

According to Lady Gaga's facialist, yes, there is a right way.

Turns out there is a right way to wash your mean mug. According to Joomee Song, a Korean Japanese skincare expert based in New York City, the secret to the entertainer's glow-worthy skin starts with skincare's first step: cleansing. While the skincare whisperer has used high-tech treatments to pamper Hollywood elites and their pores, she still says that it all starts with the basics: washing your face.

"Cleansing is one of the most important steps in skincare," she says. It's also the step that's the most misunderstood. The wrong cleanser can strip your skin of its natural oils or cause you to have even more breakouts. Worse, it could damage your skin. Here Joomee walks us through how to properly wash your face, from which products to use to how to pat dry with a towel.

1. START BY IDENTIFYING YOUR SKIN TYPE.

"The proper way to cleanse your skin starts with your understanding of the amount of oil production in your skin," Joomee says—aka how much dirt and impurities you can remove without causing dryness and/or dehydration. Most people's skin falls into one of the following categories: sensitive, dry, combination, or oily.

Sensitive or Dry—If you have sensitive skin, you'll find that your complexion turns red with a single touch, or usually after using a new product. "It means your skin lacks natural healthy oils," Joomee explains. If you're dry, you'll notice your face is tight after cleansing, or you'll see flakes on the skin. **Your cleanser type:** Hydrating oil or super-gentle milky cleansers. "These will add more oil into your skin while you cleanse," says Joomee. Instead of rinsing with water, she suggests removing the cleanser with a warm compress. "This will help keep you from stripping your own natural oils, especially if you have sensitive skin." Natural oils also give your skin an extra coating to prevent water loss.

Combination—Possibly the most complicated of skin types, this means you're oily in some areas, dry in others, and maybe sensitive in a few specific spots. Because this skin type isn't a one-cleanser-fits-all situation, Joomee suggests testing a few cleansers to see which work for you before deciding which to keep in your beauty rotation. **Your cleanser types:** milky, gel, foam. "These are ideal for combination skin as it allows your skin to have enough oil to spare," she says. Again, the key here is experimenting to see how effective a cleanser you can use without causing your pores to get dehydrated. Milky cleansers as the gentlest, gels are a little stronger, and foam are the strongest, so use them only if your skin seems to need something stronger.

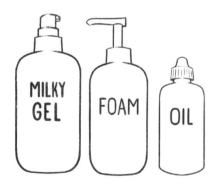

Oily—The best way to tell if you have oily skin? "Your face is covered with oil in less than one hour after cleansing," says Joomee. Still, you don't want to use anything too harsh that will overstrip your natural oils. When it comes to cleansing, the best rule of thumb is to maintain your natural hydration and oils. **Your cleanser types:** oil and gel. Use an oil cleanser first—oil traps oil, after all—and then go with a gel cleanser for a double cleanse. This one-two combination will extract impurities while also getting rid of excess oil.

2. NOW THAT YOU'VE IDENTIFIED YOUR PERFECT CLEANSER, IT'S TIME TO WASH YOUR FACE.

With warm water, splash your face to open your pores. Next, take a dime-size amount of cleanser—a little goes a long way—and use a circular motion to spread it onto your face. While there isn't a perfect method, Joomee does say that it's possible to be too harsh with your face. "Don't incorporate too much friction, which can cause irritation and inflammation," she says. "Be gentle."

After rinsing, pat your face dry instead of scrubbing your face with a towel. Being too heavy-handed can open up your pores or, worse, cause scratches. Your skin should feel balanced after cleansing, meaning if you used the right cleanser, it shouldn't feel stiff or dry, and you shouldn't feel any burning sensation. Immediately after, follow up with a toner, serum, and face cream (for more on next steps, see page 48 to read about the Korean 10-step routine).

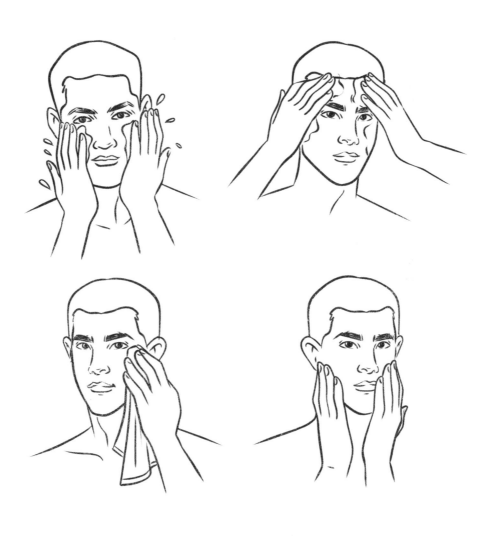

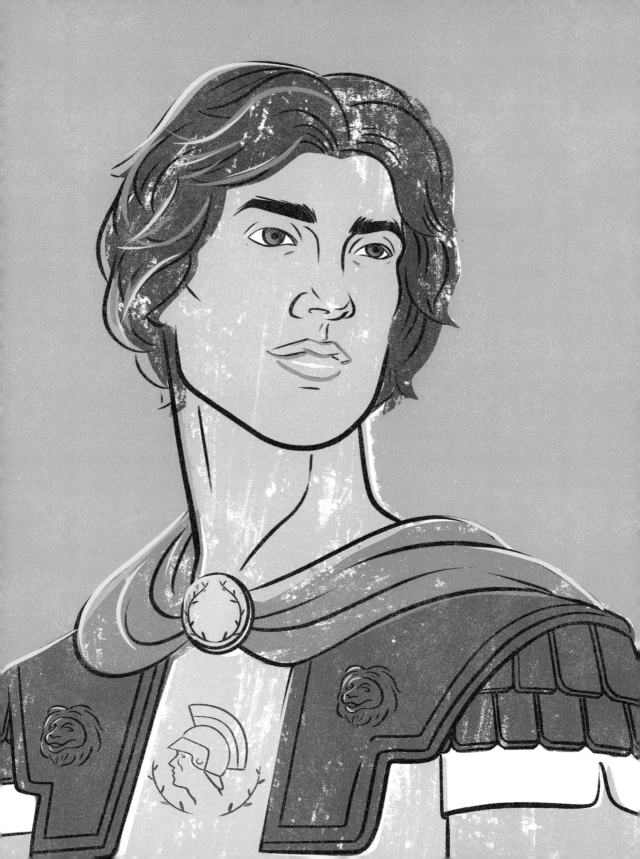

ALEXANDER THE GREAT

(356–323 BCE)

Scentual seduction.

OF ALL THE HOBBIES ALEXANDER THE GREAT COULD HAVE FIX-ated on, it was perfumes and fragrances that made his heart sing. Well, in this case, his nose. When he wasn't expanding his ever-growing empire from Europe to India, he was poring over ingredients, mixing and matching scent profiles and bottling them for use in future colognes. Who knew that one of the greatest conquerors in history was also an aroma aficionado?

"A very pleasant odor exhaled from his skin," the Greek biographer Plutarch once noted of Alexander. "There was a fragrance about his mouth and all his flesh, so that his garments were filled with it." His clothes smelled of "dry and parched regions of the world, produc[ing] the most and best spices."

When he was but a youth, Alexander III of Macedon—he was not yet anyone great—would liberally scatter frankincense around the sacred altars that lined the royal palace. He was a feckless child who didn't quite understand his parents' devotion to their religion. King Philip II and Queen Olympias worshipped the Greek gods—the queen in particular had great plans for her son, who she believed was a direct descendent of the legendary warrior Achilles. While they spoke of brawn and sheer might, Alexander was interested in other subjects, including his sense of smell.

Alexander would be scolded by his teachers for going into the royal cabinets and squandering the priceless fragrances within so liberally. One day, his tutor, Leonidas, finally rebuked him, saying, "When you have conquered the perfume-producing land then you can offer lavishly."

> *Alexander would remember this as an adult, and after he had done as his tutor instructed, he'd send Leonidas aromatic spices like passive-aggressive thank-you notes.*

When Alexander matured into a teenager, his instructor, Aristotle, the famed Greek philosopher would teach him that fragrances weren't just accoutrements for worship. They were also a measure of *arete* (Greek for "excellence") as well as *sophrosyne* ("self-restraint"). A person who understood and appreciated scents was someone who would be able to be "balanced and logical," as well as what Aristotle described as "intellectual"—all signs of a great leader.

From then on, Alexander would use smell as his secret weapon: scents would calm him in times of high stress and seep into his mind, unlocking sweet memories from childhood while he was away from home. As much as he was an ambitious king, he was also one who relied on his senses as well as his intellect to survive.

> *At the time, spices that were favorable to Aphrodite, the goddess of love, were favorable to rulers. These included frankincense, myrrh, costus root, cassia, cinnamon, and bay laurel—the last of which was often associated with the god Apollo.*

With every country he'd enter, Alexander brought a man named Theophrastus—who would later become known as the Greek "father of botany"—an essential member of Alexander's executive team. The botanist would help identify exotic aromatic plants and seeds for him. Later, he'd use them to establish Greece's first botanical gardens, one of the greatest of the time period, and write the first book about odors, titled *De Odoribus (Concerning Odors)*.

Alexander's military and olfactory tour from the deserts of Egypt to the mountains of India to the historic grounds of the Persian Empire eventually ended in Babylon. There, he developed a fever, and died at the late King Nebuchadnezzar's palace at the age of thirty-two. He never made it back to his childhood home in Macedon, but during the last days of his life, he was able to travel space and time with each whiff of essential oils, every spray of cologne bringing back memories of his youth and his journeys.

While this Grecian is known as one of history's greatest military minds, he is also one of the forefathers of fragrances, from the mixing and matching of various notes to the chronicling of scent profiles with his team to the process of bottling them en masse. Of course, other peoples, including the Egyptians, Indians, and Persians, had been using essential oils for years. But it was through Alexander's initiatives that the use of fragrance became normalized on a mass scale. As a man who bottled up his feels and wore them on his sleeves, he created and arguably jump-started a global fragrance trade that still thrives today. And perhaps he was the first to fully grasp the power of smell—the way it allows for a specific moment of history, or even a person, to return to an exact moment. Scent has that ability . . . to allow us to travel back in time for a conversation with a beloved, to observe that fond memory again, feel an emotion from yesterday—if even for just a second.

THE NOSE KNOWS: A GUIDE TO SCENT

What's the difference between perfumes, colognes, and everything else?

Smells. Historically, fragrances have not been gendered. It was only at the turn of the twentieth century that specific types of scents began to be marketed toward men (cologne) and women (perfume). Fast-forward to today, and we're a culture obsessed with fragrances. Whether it's a spritz from a fashion house or a splash from a Brooklyn indie brand, scents are indicators of a person's own personality. Better yet, there are now new genderless fragrance brands. With so many fragrances to choose from, where do you start?

With your nose, of course! First, sniff around: Are you more of a floral person? Into citruses, or more about woodsy notes?

Once you discover what you're drawn to, take a look at concentration levels. Fragrances are a blend of synthetic and natural oils, diluted with alcohols to not only stabilize the formula but act as a preservative. Not all of these scents are created equal.

The higher the concentration, the longer the fragrance will last. Pure perfumes, for instance, contain 20 to 30 percent perfume oil, and should last from day to night. But often, these are not only more expensive, but too strong for the average consumer. At right is a graph of how long fragrances last, by their concentration and classification.

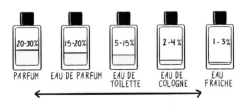

FRAGRANCE CONCENTRATION GUIDE

| 20-30% | 15-20% | 5-15% | 2-4% | 1-3% |

PARFUM   EAU DE PARFUM   EAU DE TOILETTE   EAU DE COLOGNE   EAU FRAICHE

LASTS UP TO 8HRS   LASTS LESS THAN 2HRS

The best method of spritzing yourself? Keep in mind that less is more. Choose a pulse point on your body and spritz there; the heat emitted at that spot will slowly create a cloud of beautiful, invisible vapor over time. Your pulse points may include the radial pulses on the insides of your wrists, the carotid pulses on your neck, the brachial pulses under your elbows, or even popliteal pulse at the backs of the knees. Wherever you choose for your scent, spritz that one part and no others. The last thing you need is to become a walking migraine-inducing agent! *No one*—and we mean *no one*—appreciates anyone who smells a little too strongly of any fragrance, no matter how good it may be.

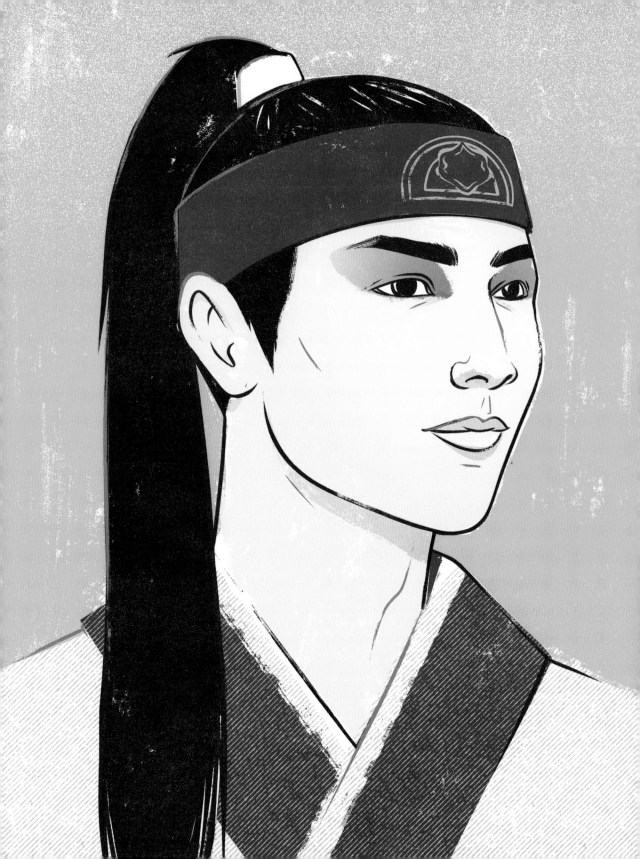

HWARANG

The "Flower Boy" warriors of the sixth century.

SOUTH KOREA IS NOW KNOWN AS THE BEAUTY CAPITAL OF THE universe, and its men hold the title of world's biggest cosmetics consumers. Korean men glisten and glow, their complexions plumped and hydrated, as if serums pump through their very veins. But to understand why Korean men today care so much about their aesthetics, we must look to Korea's sixth-century Silla Dynasty, and to the hwarang. The *hwarang*—which roughly translates to "flower boys"—weren't only some of the fiercest weapons-wielding, martial arts–practicing assassins in Asia. They would become legendary for their fight *and* their faces. Aesthetics, and the spirituality behind beautifying, were paramount to their ability to defend their kingdom for over two centuries . . . and to lead the way for generations of Korean beauty boys to come.

Like all the Silla, the hwarang were devout followers of Maitreya, the future Buddha. Ancient texts say he manifested into human form to live among mortals as a lean, teenage pretty boy before the nation of Silla was formed. It was said that his look was so striking, all were awed by his presence. The kingdom of Silla awaited his return on Earth as Christians await the return of Christ: it is foretold that he'll return to save humanity. Legend has it that when Maitreya's physical form died, his spirit reincarnated into Silla's soil to be reborn in the physical form of young men who resembled him. That meant that any young man in the aristocracy who happened to be pretty could also very well be Maitreya incarnate. Talk about winning the genetic—and spiritual—lottery!

But Silla's wily king Jinheung had big plans for those fated pretty boys. For years, the king had been testing his allies' patience, slowly plotting to take over the entire Korean peninsula. The Korean nation had been split into three kingdoms for centuries at that point: Baekje in the west, Goguryeo in the north, and Silla, which occupied land to the east. King Jinheung had helped the Baekje reclaim their land from the Goguryeo, but quickly turned on the Baekje right after, breaking a sacred 120-year alliance. At the end of the war between Baekje and Silla, one that was years-long and tireless, Silla was left as vulnerable as ever. In his final days, King Jinheung was paralyzed by fear and consumed by paranoia. He knew his enemies were thirsty for revenge, and were after his people's complete downfall.

To keep his enemies at bay and his kingdom alive for centuries to come, King Jinheung needed power that none of his enemies had. He needed something supernatural, that Big Buddha Energy. Silla's pretty boys were the only ones who could deliver, he thought. After all, the prettier the boy, the closer to god—and these men were packing!

King Jinheung searched for every beautiful boy throughout the kingdom who came from true bone status.[1] The search was methodical and swift (like, a few months swift!), and a year after his hunt began, in 576 CE, the hwarang was implemented as an official arm of Silla's military. As detailed in the *Samguk Yusa,* a historic Korean record, these young men would immediately go through rigorous training that not only stripped them from their families, but demanded their excellence in all things physical, emotional, and spiritual.

The hwarang trainees mastered martial arts, swordfighting, and hwarangdo (a specific style of martial arts created for the hwarang by Silla monks), horsemanship, stone throwing, archery, and javelin, as well as perfecting song and dance and memorizing religious texts. These "soft" skills allowed the men to become well-rounded warriors. Instilled with great discipline, each was also indoctrinated with Taoist, shamanist, and Buddhist teachings. Many became so devout that they even believed they'd encounter Maitreya before they died.

And in true Maitreya fashion, it's believed that the boys perfected their appearances as well—the closer they resembled Maitreya, the closer they would be to divinity. "They selected the handsome boys of the nobility and adorned them, powdering their faces and calling them Hwarang," wrote an envoy for the Tang dynasty. "The people of the country all respected and supported them."

---

1. True bone status comes from Silla's caste system, called the "bone-rank system." The system ranked all people who lived within Silla society, segregating them based on their proximity to royal blood. "Sacred bone" meant you were part of the royal family. "True bone" indicated you were aristocratic. Everyone else was a part of the head ranks from sixth, fifth, and fourth, where sixth was the highest.

> *Unfortunately, there exists no information on the specific makeup they used, but we can look to the Chinese Tang dynasty, whom the Silla were influenced by, and make an educated guess. In historic texts, the Chinese detail face powder ingredients as being made of (lethal) lead, rice, and clamshell powder mixed together to create a thick, pearly foundation.*

In addition to face powder, modern scholars believe the hwarang would have used red eyeshadow to distinguish themselves as elite warriors, as well as appearing more intimidating during battle.

> *The red dye the hwarang may have used on their eyes would have been created from safflower and red lily, and was also used by Chinese royals as a cheek, eye, and lip stain.*

Per the time period, their long hair may have also been hydrated with oil produced from apricot seeds and peach kernels (*way* fancier than St. Ives). Some hwarang are also depicted with pierced ears and beautiful clothing—when you're already fancy, what's a little more?

When the hwarang officially made their debut, they became overnight sensations. Precursors to boy bands like NCT 127, The Boyz, or even BTS, who are now worldwide heartthrobs, they had tongues wagging all the way from Silla to China. As King Jinheung had once predicted, his enemies would one day attack Silla. In the midsummer of 660 CE, the Baekje launched an attack against the Silla, which would become known as the famous Battle of Hwangsanbeol. But the hwarang, fighting together with the Tang army, would prevail against the Baekje, sending the enemy cowering. For over three hundred years, the hwarang would defend their borders from outsiders—without smudging their eyeshadow—until they, too, were overthrown by another power. In 935 CE, they surrendered in defeat to Korea's last dynasty, the Goryeo, which would go on to unify the entire Korean peninsula. Though the hwarang were dissolved by the new power, their legacy wasn't completely erased: the Goryeo government took pride in Silla's past, and made attempts to celebrate hwarang history over the years.

To this day, no one can deny how mystical and magical these "flower boy" warriors were. In contemporary Korea, the hwarang are still extolled for their bravery and celebrated for their beauty, and South Korea's men's beauty business leads the way for innovations around the world. Korean pop culture celebrates men's beauty, from TV shows like OnStyle's *Lipstick Prince,* a program that features male K-pop idols learning about makeup and putting cosmetics on each other, to K-dramas like 2016's popular *Hwarang: The Poet Warrior Youth,* which cast K-pop's biggest names and prettiest faces in the role of warriors, from BTS's V to SHINee's Minho. These are only some of South Korea's contemporary flower boys, who some shamanists would argue possess the hwarang spirit, alive and well (and pretty!).

Smoldering, sultry, sexy, and *fierce*. There's a reason the hwarang would use eye pigments as a means of instilling fear on and off the battlefield. Of course, the Koreans weren't the first to use eyeshadows. Eyeshadow dates back to Ancient Egypt, with the use of smudged kohl. (Read more about how to Rule Over Your Eyeliner on page 28.) The use of eye makeup is even documented in the Old Testament! Ezekiel 23:40: "They even sent messengers for men who came from far away, and when they arrived you bathed yourself for them, applied eye makeup and put on your jewelry." While in ancient times there were a limited number of colors to choose from, in today's vibrant world, there's every shade under the sun. That means you can change up your look depending on what kind of mood you're in. Whether you want a natural look for daytime or a bold look for TikTok, eyeshadow is a great way to not only bring dimension to your eyes, but to make them stand out.

Having worked with the likes of Meghan Markle (for her wedding!), Bella Hadid, Gemma Chan, Saoirse Ronan, Priyanka Chopra, and others, celebrity makeup artist Daniel Martin is one of Hollywood's greatest beauty advisors. Read on for his step-by-step on how to make your lids stand out and sparkle.

1. A PRIMER ON PRIMER.

Your face produces oils. So do your eyelids. To lock down eyeshadow so it'll last longer, you want a nice base—for that, you need a primer. For those of you who don't know what that is, primer is a product that locks makeup onto your skin. Just like face primers that prevent foundation from sliding off, eye primers hold on to eyeshadow. Daniel suggests taking an eyeshadow brush, painting your lids with primer, then adding setting powder. The powder creates a seal over the eyeshadow so your natural oils don't melt it away.

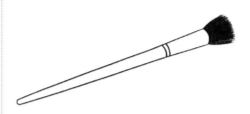

2. TOOLS OF THE TRADE.

Whether you're a beginner or a pro, Daniel says there's one brush everyone needs to own: a smudger. A smudger brush has dome-shaped bristles that allow you to layer eyeshadows, create smokiness, or apply colors.

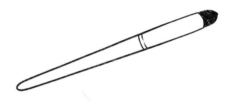

3. CREAMS, LIQUIDS, OR POWDERS?

When it comes to eyeshadows, one type isn't better than another. But some *are* easier to use. Powders are probably best for beginners, as powder allows for mistakes, wipes off easily, and can be layered. Creams are versatile as well and can be smudged onto your lids with your fingers.

> **PRO TIP:** Make sure the cream eyeshadow of your choosing doesn't melt. You can achieve this through powder setting or choosing water-resistant formulas. Otherwise on hot or humid days, there can be makeup running down your face.

Finally, there are liquid eyeshadows, which often come in a tube with a doe-foot applicator included, like lip gloss. Liquid shadow dries quickly, so you'll want to practice using it so you know exactly how much time you have to apply.

4. LAY OF THE LAND.
How much of your eyelid should you coat with shadow? For monolids (or hooded eyelids), Martin says to use your finger as a guide: take your ring finger and tap it upwards until you find your eye socket. "It helps set the guide because you can see where it hits the bone." If you have double eyelids, paint them with shadow up to the crease.

5. SHAPE AND LAYER.
"Eyeshadows are great because you can really create dimension and shape to your eyes," Martin says. When you're ready to apply, start with a more neutral color to set the foundation. Then take a darker brown or black and use it to paint in the eyeline. From there, paint outward and upward to create an almond shape. Add colors of your choice, whether a dramatic pop of color or something more subdued, directly to the lids.

> **PRO TIP:** "I take a vibrant color and paint it in the middle of the eyelid, then brush up. No need to blend—it allows the eye to really hold that specific shade."

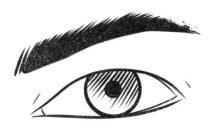

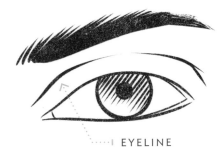

EYELINE

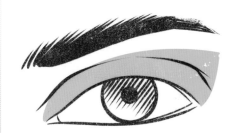

Is it 10 steps or 100? Soko Glam's Charlotte Cho breaks it down.

If you haven't heard of Korean beauty, well, brace yourself. Korean beauty, or K-beauty for short, is for those *serious* about getting their best glow. In the past decade, South Korea has become the world's beauty mecca, thanks to its innovative products that are light-years ahead of the rest. It's where sheet masks and snail mucin were made popular, where pimple patches were normalized. And it only helped that Korean celebrities became the global ambassadors of K-beauty. Their bouncy skin, juicy complexions, and flawless faces are proof that Koreans know what they're doing.

Or so says Charlotte Cho, cofounder and aesthetician behind Soko Glam, the Korean beauty site that offers the best of Korean beauty products. The entrepreneur is behind the infamous "10-Step Korean Skin Care Routine" interview that went viral in *Elle* back in 2012 and changed the beauty world forever. "The article compelled people to take the steps literally," Charlotte says in retrospect. Ultimately, Charlotte explains, the ten steps are not about using literally ten different products all together. "It's about having the knowledge to understand what products and steps are right for you to achieve your skin goals," she says. "In Korea, the practice of taking care of your skin begins at an early age, like basic hygiene practices. The more time you invest in taking care of your skin and understanding what you are using, the better the results."

TL;DR: Don't be deterred by the idea of having to do each step or use ten products in one night! Charlotte takes you through each one in the order in which they should be applied, but keep in mind that you should pick and choose which steps your skin needs on any given day.

Warning: Applying a combination of the following will give your skin some serious glow.

1. OIL CLEANSE.

It's the first step in your "double cleanse" method. Don't let the "oil" in the name deter you—this step works for all skin types, including those that are acne-prone or oily. An oil-based product breaks down oil-based impurities such as makeup and SPF.

2. WATER CLEANSE.

The second step in your double cleanse method helps you get rid of anything left over. Water-based cleansers break down water-based debris such as dirt and sweat, and typically come in foam formulas. Charlotte recommends doing a double cleanse both morning and night!

3. EXFOLIATE.

This is a step you can do weekly. Use a chemical-based exfoliator that includes an ingredient like alpha-hydroxy acids (AHAs), which will penetrate skin and clean deep in your pores.

> AHAs unglue dead skin cells that may not break away otherwise. Your skin is so efficient, it holds skin cells together like superglue! While this is amazing for protecting your skin, if you produce too many cells, they can be difficult to shed and will begin to clog your pores. Use this as a toning step or after, if your toner is acid-free.

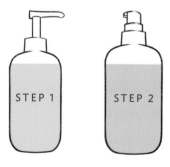

STEP 1   STEP 2

If you want an extra-buffed feeling, you can use a mechanical exfoliant like a sugar scrub instead, to slough off anything extra that may still be hanging on to the exterior layer of your skin.

4. TONE.
Do this after you cleanse (or exfoliate, if you've chosen to do that step today). A lot of toner formulas of the past were very astringent and left faces "squeaky clean," but that's beginning to change, especially as Western companies take cues from Korean ones. Korean toners focus on hydrating the skin, prepping it to better absorb the other products in your skincare routine. (If you want to include a sheet mask in your routine right now, skip to step 7!)

5. ESSENCE.
After you tone, your skin is prepared for essence, which is typically a liquid formula that's made with ingredients that help make your skin look less dull and brighten your complexion by encouraging skin cells to regenerate.

6. AMPOULE.
This is like a denser, slicker version of essence that's supercharged with ingredients that help address signs of skin damage, whether it's plumping fine lines by making sure skin is properly hydrated or reducing the appearance of hyperpigmentation through skin renewal.

7. SHEET MASKS.
These are perhaps the most recognizable step in Korean skincare regimens. You can use them once or twice a week. As the name suggests, a sheet mask is a thin cotton or gel sheet that you wear for about 15 minutes. Typically, they've been soaked in serums and essences, which means you don't need to apply any extra products that day. Many sheet masks are specially formulated to treat a particular skin concern, ranging from acne to dryness and much more.

8. EYE CREAM.
The skin around the eyes is especially delicate, so you want to use something richer here than you do on the rest of your face. Use a tapping

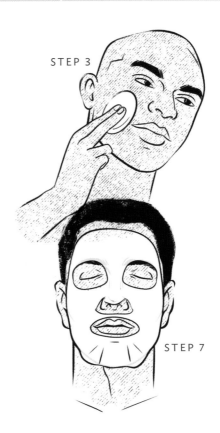

STEP 3

STEP 7

motion to apply the cream, as opposed to a rubbing motion, to avoid stretching the skin, which could lead to wrinkles down the road.

9. MOISTURIZER.
A good moisturizer is one that works to penetrate into the skin and hydrate at a deeper level. At night, you can substitute a sleeping mask, a product that you use overnight to really seep into your pores. Use a sleeping mask on nights when you feel extra dry; layer it onto your skin as a last step and wash it off in the morning.

10. SUNSCREEN.
Arguably the most important step in your routine, daily SPF use is vital, as it protects your skin from harmful UVA and UVB rays, which can lead to hyperpigmentation, wrinkles, and other signs of aging, as well as cause skin cancer.

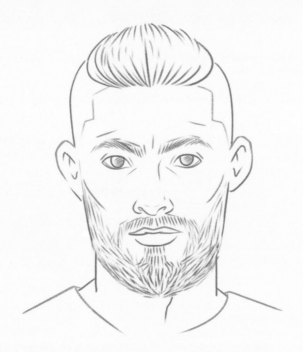

VIKINGS

(700-900 CE)

Beauty and the brawn.

I T ' S W E L L D O C U M E N T E D T H A T T H E V I K I N G S W E R E S E X Y A F.
Towering, brawny, and chiseled, sure—but these men worked hard at their grooming, too.
So serious were they about their attractive appearances, each Viking carried a custom-made
beauty kit (one of the earliest forms of dopp kits!) tucked neatly into their belts next to their
axes and swords—these fierce warriors were always ready to shine on the spot.

> *These kits included custom combs for both hair and beards, ear picks to
> remove wax, and tweezers to pluck stray hairs from their eyebrows.*

Most European hygiene during this time period was appalling at best. Anglo-Saxons bathed
only a few times a year, under the belief that dirt was good for protecting the skin from
diseases and preventing them from entering the body. There were some religious aspects

to this as well, with some Christians viewing bathing as an act of sinful vanity. Whatever the case, you can only imagine just how putrid most of these Europeans must have been.

Their Nordic neighbors, on the other hand, were squeaky clean. For a single day each week, they stopped everything to soak in a bath. The Old Norse word for "Saturday" was *laugardagr,* which directly translates as "bathing day."

On *laugardagr,* they dunked themselves into hot springs (rich with natural sulfur that helped heal wounded skin), scrubbing their bodies, buffing their faces, and washing their hair with lye-and-vegetable-oil soap. After their extensive bathing process, they'd brush their hair until it had a nice sheen. Each man had his own personalized comb carved out of expensive bone, antler, wood, and/or ivory. Particular care was given to their locks, as a Viking's hair was a means to display one's class and a representation of one's virility and masculinity. The longer the hair, the more strapping the person, whether noble or warrior. So important was hair for the Vikings that it was against the law to cut a man's hair short without his consent. So sacred were these locks that warriors would tie their hair back in battle to ensure that blood wouldn't soak in.

But even more important than their hair were their beards. Facial hair was grown in imitation of Norse gods like Thor, who was depicted with a curled mustache and a long, thick beard. To get a supple, bushy, soft beard, Viking men didn't use shampoo, which would strip their strands of important natural oils and make the texture feel bristly and dehydrated. Instead, Vikings kept their beards soft with a special oil made of goat fat and beechwood ash. The more outré would dye their beards red or blond with lye soap, which had bleaching properties said to help with the coloring process. Beyond being a fashion choice, coloring the hair could have also marked a Viking's tribal identity.

However, these Viking men's striking looks didn't settle well with their neighbors. The English monk and reporter John of Wallingford recorded how hopeless men of the time felt next to their more attractive northern neighbors: "In the habit of combing their hair every day, to bathe every Saturday, to change their clothes frequently and to draw attention to themselves by means of many such frivolous whims . . . they sieged the married women's virtue and persuaded the daughters of even noble men to become their mistresses." (Of course, yet another problematic example of the objectification of women throughout history.)

The wandering Vikings eventually settled in places like Northern England, Iceland, and Greenland, or remained in Scandinavia, after retiring from their pirate professions. Sadly, stink won out, as Christianity became more influential. Centuries later, Vikings would be depicted as savages, gruff men who wore horns on their helmets and were only obsessed with physical power. But the Viking were just as fearless when it came to beauty as to brawn—they knew their aesthetics were just as mighty as any of their other weapons, that a hairpin could be as mighty as a sword.

If you've passed puberty, you've probably had to reach for a razor at some point, if not daily. Whether it's your underarms, chest hair, nether regions, or face, shaving can get complicated—and messy. It's no wonder men throughout the centuries have gone to experts to get a shave. But in our modern world, there are plenty of products—and really good razors!—to get you the perfect shave without a barber.

Here's a list of the tools you'll need to shave anywhere and a step-by-step guide on how to do it.

- Fresh razor
- Shaving cream or gel (creams are thicker, gels foam with water—take your pick!)
- Beard oil
- Grooming scissors (if you have long whiskers)
- Post-shave balm

1. CLEANSE AND EXFOLIATE.

As in any part of skincare, you want to ensure your skin is clean. This will help prevent ingrown hairs, or worse—infection. Though the latter is really rare, it can still happen if you shave unclean skin.

2. OIL CHANGE.

The best way to prep the hair to be shaved is to soften it first with an oil. A beard oil can also act as a protective barrier between your skin and the razor, helping to prevent cuts. Once applied, allow the oil to sit on your hair for a good 5 minutes before putting on shaving cream.

3. FOAM TOWN HERO.

Shaving creams have been used forever because they really do work. The product lathers and foams into a beautiful texture to provide moisture and protection to your skin, and allows your razor to glide effortlessly. After applying your shaving cream, you can let it sit on top of your hair for a few moments; let it soak through for a closer shave.

4. WITH THE GRAIN OR AGAINST?

There are two camps: those who shave with the grain, and those who shave against the grain. The latter are masochists (that, or they have skin made of steel!). Yes, you'll get a closer shave going against the grain, but you'll probably irritate your skin in the process. If you're in for the easiest shave, shaving with the grain of your hair growth makes for the most harmonious experience. Don't know which way your hair's growing? Take your fingers and lightly run it across your skin as if you're shaving. If there's little to no resistance to your fingertips, you're definitely with the grain. If it's prickly and feels like petting your cat the wrong way, you're going against the grain. If you can't tell, let the hair grow just a little bit more and then try again. After determining this, take your blade and gently glide it onto your skin. After shaving your hair, gently pat the excess hair into your sink and shave until your desired facial hair length.

5. AFTERCARE

Razor bumps, burns, cuts—they all happen. Pain comes with the territory. When they do, head toward your medicine cabinet. Gently pat on antiseptic (it's okay to scream!) and put a Band-Aid on if you're bleeding. For your face, you'll want to apply aftershave. Don't have a post-shave balm? It's cool! Go for your toner and moisturizer, and allow them to soothe your skin. After all, hallelu, it just went through a lot!

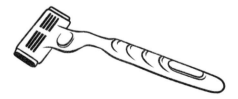

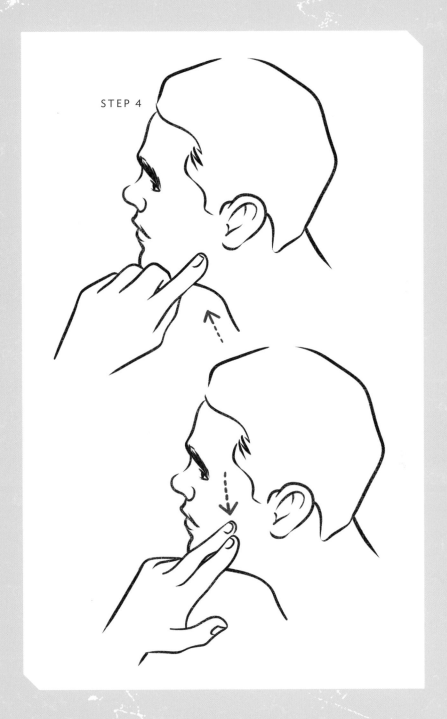

STEP 4

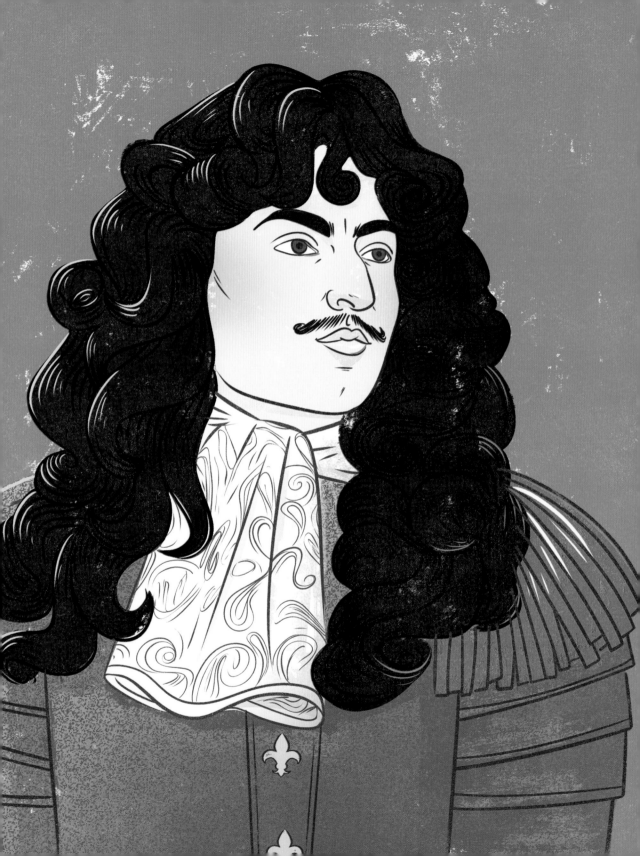

KING LOUIS XIV

(1 6 3 8 - 1 7 1 5)

The Emperor's new wig.

"KING LOUIS XIV IS FLAWLESS."

"I hear his hair's insured for $10,000."

Okay, these are lines from 2004's *Mean Girls,* but they might as well be from Voltaire. Because when it comes to trendsetting ways, there was no one greater than the HBIC to *all* pretty boys himself, King Louis XIV, the Regina George of the seventeenth century. This king would influence fashionistas for centuries to come.

Aptly nicknamed "the Sun King," everything—and everyone—revolved around Louis's opulent orbit. Case in point: That one time he made wigs into the hottest accessory across all of Europe (kind of like when Regina George started a trend by wearing a tank top with cutouts on her boobs). That's how fly King Louis XIV was.

Golden gowns? Yes, God. Sparkly heels? Sickening. Hip-grazing wigs? Say no more.

It was the 1600s, and long, flowy hair was a status symbol—as it did for the Vikings, hair stood for health, wealth, and virility. And sex appeal. Back when the king's hair was still thick and curly, it had a feathery, diaphanous texture with a sheen that was *made* for a Pantene commercial. France became obsessed with the young king's luscious locks. Iconic portraits of him and his full head of hair hung in the hallways of his royal court and throughout the land.

At seventeen years old, King Louis XIV declared that wigs were cool. At the time, they were seen as frumpy, scratchy contraptions fit only for the clumsy, diseased, or old. Not chic, especially not for a royal. It was peculiar when the teenage king requested one . . . but his own hair was thinning out and shedding.

This was the golden age of syphilis, the STI that refused to go away. One of its many side effects—other than death—was hair loss. While the palace staff certainly speculated that the teenaged king was liberally practicing free love, as influential young men were wont to do, whether he actually carried the venereal disease is still unknown.

But with his hair falling out in clumps, Louis was left hanging on to two choices: he could either go bald, or sport false hair. The decision was clear. He was the Sun King, after all, and such a formidable figure needed a larger-than-life persona to match his name. And as a petite man (standing a grand 5 feet, 3 inches), a big, bold, beautiful set of hair (and later, tall heels) could provide him with additional, even more regal height.

In a matter of days, the course of male beauty standards would change forever. The king requested that France's most prominent wigmaker, Georges Binet, create an original hair-piece—and an entirely new aesthetic—for him. Binet was prominent for owning one of the most popular wig shops in Paris. (Think of him as the seventeenth-century version of the modern-day Insta-famous hairstylist Chris Appleton, the man behind many of Kim Kardashian's looks.)

Binet immediately rolled up his sleeves and set out on a quest to discover the best hair around. After searching far and wide, he discovered exceptionally fine, healthy hair in the northern part of France, among the Normans, who came from Viking lineage. He paid Norman women to shear their locks. He also kept them on retainer to grow their hair, and paid them extra to keep their heads covered to protect the hair from damage. Needless to say, Binet spared no expense. "I would strip every head in the kingdom bald in order to adorn that of his majesty," he later said.

After retrieving hundreds of pounds of hair, the wigmaker went to work designing the king's new look. It would have to be not only luxe but elegant, giving height as well as splendor and grace. The final product was a piece made from ten full heads' worth of human hair and took three months to complete. It was called a "full bottom" wig, a mid-part style with lavish curls that grazed the middle back, while both halves were shaped into peaks for extreme volume.

When Louis finally debuted his new look, his kingdom was not ready. They snatched wigs—literally. Wigs flew off of the shelves as the kingdom gasped in collective shock and awe. Overnight, the wig was resurrected from the depths of fashion hell and deemed a must-have accessory. Royals flocked to buy their own, some even going into debt in their attempts to fit in. It wasn't just about purchasing a single wig, which went for around 150 livres (approximately $7,500 today), either: The real cost came in having to purchase multiples and in paying for wig maintenance.

Wigmakers charged a heavy fee for the labor-extensive upkeep of their products. Their services included washing, styling, and primping the wigs. The process started with collecting the wigs, then washing away excess oils, dirt, and sweat, drying them, and then carefully curling and restyling them. The final touches came in the form of perfume and powders to keep the curls intact and smelling pleasant.

Wigmakers became so in demand, they had difficulties keeping up with orders. In Paris, the number of wigmakers went from just a couple throughout the city to two hundred the next year. By 1673, the number had skyrocketed to 835. So big was business that Le Havre, a small city with a population of only 18,000, had twenty-nine wigmakers in total. Soon, a wigmakers guild was established to ensure that all wigs being made met an excellent standard.

The king would build an entire wing at Versailles dedicated to wigs. The rooms lined up his thousands of wigs for all occasions, with a handful of staffers whose sole role was maintaining them full-time.

The trend didn't stay inside the confines of France. Not when you were the Regina George of Europe! When England's King Charles II, Louis's cousin, visited France, he left with a new appreciation for wigs and brought the trend back to Britain. Soon enough, all of Britain followed suit, with everyone form royals to commoners sporting wigs. In only a decade, you couldn't step inside a European country without finding a man in a wig.

The king capitalized on his influence, up-charging wigs and other items from fashion to textiles, catapulting businesses into fashion and beauty empires. France's entire economy thrived under the sale of luxury goods, becoming Europe's biggest exporter. "Fashions were to France what the mines of Peru were to Spain," the king's finance minister, Jean-Baptiste Colbert, once said. Under King Louis XIV's reign, France became an economic powerhouse with a legacy for storied beauty and fashion brands that has persisted through to the present.

What was a necessity to hide baldness became a defining feature of men's aesthetics throughout the seventeenth century. After Louis died in 1715, wigs thrived for close to another century, until the French Revolution, when everything perceived as excessive was frowned upon (RIP, Marie-Antoinette). These days, trends might be a certain sneaker, a bag, or a makeup palette—still, we hide behind our beauty and fashion purchases in the hopes that they will gain us a share of perceived power. That sentiment has never changed throughout history. But in our modern times, we also talk about how embracing who you already are can be transformative. An individual who has their own sense of style and beautifies for themselves? Now *that's* fetch.

Just say oui *to wigs.*

Ancient civilizations—from the Egyptians to societies in the Middle East to East Asians—have rocked wigs for centuries for a variety of reasons, whether out of practicality or fashion or as a class signifier. But it was King Louis XIV who turned wigs into a European must-have. Of course, Louis's wigs were extremely heavy (and, dare we say, itchy and hot), as their lengths would stretch to three-quarters of the Sun King's stature.

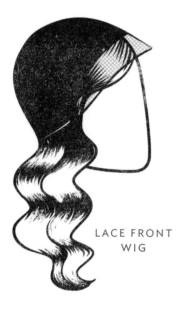

LACE FRONT
WIG

Today, wigs are just as popular—and thankfully, much lighter—and are again being worn daily or as an embellishment. To get all the hairy details of finding your own perfect wig, we sought out help from celebrity hairstylist David Lopez, whose clients include Ashley Graham, Chrissy Teigen, and Hailey Bieber. According to Lopez, it all comes down to the look you're going for: bright and expressive, more natural, or a statement piece. Here, we wig out with Lopez, who explains *all* the hair secrets you need to know before starting this journey.

1. WHAT'S THE OCCASION?

First things first: Identify where you're heading out to and also how real you need the wig to look. "That will definitely identify how much money you're going to invest in a potential wig," Lopez says. If it's for one single night, it's probably safe to purchase an affordable synthetic wig. Need it more for multiple uses, or to perform in? Perhaps try a wig made of real hair, which is more of an investment. Be forewarned: "The more realistic you need it to be, the more money you're going to spend," Lopez says.

2. SYNTHETIC VERSUS REAL.

Just because it's synthetic hair doesn't mean it isn't beautiful. "There are really amazing synthetics that are only $35—but I've never spent more than $60 [on a synthetic]," Lopez says. A real benefit of synthetic wigs is that they're always prestyled. So for the person who isn't a pro at styling longer hair or doesn't have the time, synthetic is the way to go. "The hairline is plucked, it already looks realistic, and you can really wear it out without breaking the bank," he says. It's also great for newbies who want to try out their first wigs without commitment. But there are downsides. "Synthetics can look really shiny and won't behave like human hair." Upkeep is also difficult—"It gets a little ratty." Human hair wigs, sold as what are called "blanks," are great for those who like to change hairstyles or want versatility. Before using a human hair wig, though, you'll first have to pluck the hairs to create a realistic hairline. You'll also have to pay much more for upkeep, which includes tweezing, washing, conditioning, and drying. Expect to spend anywhere from $100 to thousands, depending on the length. "You can definitely spend more than $60 on a synthetic wig if it's being customized for you or very elaborate," he says. "For the blanks, most people won't buy them because they're not able to customize like a hairstylist."

Instead, they'll buy human hair wigs that have been customized, which will cost you around $500 and up."

3. CAP IT OFF.

Most people can't wear a wig without a wig cap. "For wigs to lay as flat as possible, you want to make your own hair as flat as possible," Lopez says. You'll want to find a cap that matches your skin tone or foundation. If you can't find one in your exact shade, use foundation. "I'll rub it over my wig cap so it becomes the same color or a little bit lighter than my skin," he says. That final touch will allow the wig to look all the more natural, when you see "skin" through the wig's part. If you have long hair, you can braid it down into a low ponytail, split it, and pin the ends to the sides of your head.

4. A LACE AGAINST TIME.

Full lace vs. lace front, what's the difference? The former is when hair is woven into a lace cap. This provides ventilation as well as ease of moving the hair every which way. The latter is laced in the front but fully enclosed in the back, and the hair is attached to a hairpiece that resembles your natural scalp. The hair is sewn on top of the crown and can only be styled in one or two ways. Full laces are much more expensive than lace-front wigs because of their versatility, but Lopez says the latter is a great option as it "blends with your natural hairline better."

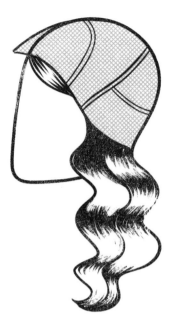

either a filled sink or a big bowl of warm water and just a regular shampoo."

PRO TIP: Go cheap. "Just get a really inexpensive drugstore shampoo; that's totally fine," says Lopez.

PRO TIP: Lace tape. "It's like theatrical tape," says Lopez. "You stick the lace to it so then you can fully pull your hair up to style— your wig will stay 'glued' to your head." You can also quite literally use wig glue as well. Another great product? Any heavy-hold hairspray. "Spray it to your hairline. Let it get tacky, spray it again and then you push the wig down and it's held there."

---

5. WASH, RINSE, REPEAT.

Both synthetic *and* real wigs need to be washed. For synthetic, "I would suggest putting it into

After placing it in warm water, detangle it, then dunk it like you're doing a delicate wash. After shampooing, rinse under cool water. If you use glue, use alcohol or acetone to remove the excess glue from the lace. "Always air-dry!" For real wigs, wash as you would real hair, with shampoo, conditioner, the works. But be gentle—real wigs are sensitive. If you want to extend its use, Lopez suggests applying a hair mask overnight. "I do use some restorative masks that have proteins or keratins to rebuild the coating." The next morning, wash the wig, put it on a wig block, air-dry, and style with a curling iron or flat iron.

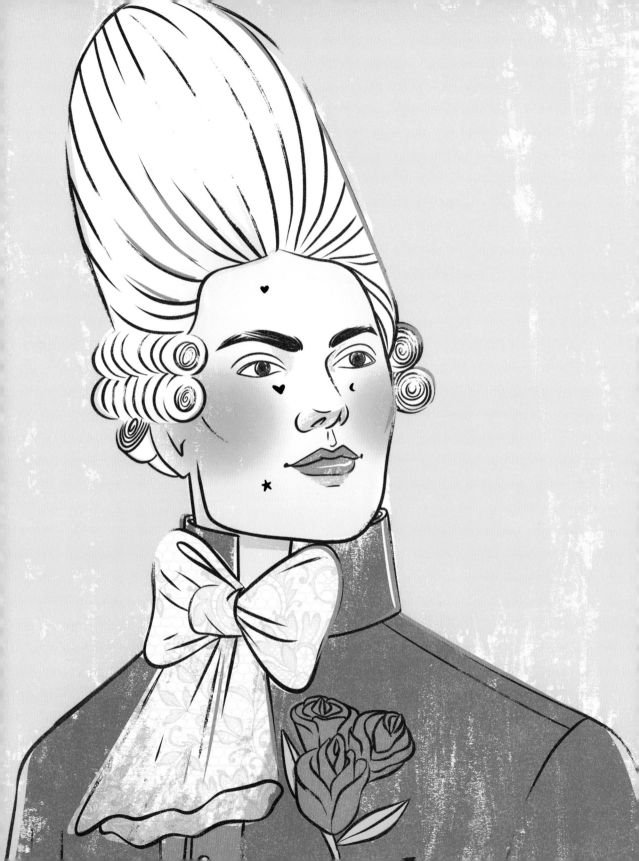

MACARONI

(1 7 6 0 s - 1 8 0 0 s)

The "Gen Z" of eighteenth-century Great Britain.

IF MASCULINITY IS FRAGILE IN OUR MODERN ERA, IT MIGHT have been worse in mid-1700s Great Britain. It was then that stodgy conservatives (ahem, the boomers of their day) were so pressed over a group of men who pushed the boundaries of male expression that they actively—and obsessively—set out to destroy them. Mind you, the older generation was still accustomed to tradition, which focused on the working class and conservative values. Their biggest grievance? That these fabulous men dared to celebrate their outward appearances by baking their faces, fluffing their hair, and seasoning their outfits *without* asking for permission. "There is indeed a kind of animal, neither male nor female, a thing of the neuter gender lately started up among us," a publication at the time wrote about them. These men were facetiously given the nickname "Macaroni" to poke fun at their predilections for all things foreign and ornate, from fashions to makeup to food, including love for the elbow noodle in question. (For years, the British had perceived the Italians as being overly foppish, outlandish, and odd. *Town and Country Magazine,* published March 1772, explained the craze: "The Italians are extremely fond of a dish they call Macaroni, composed of a kind of paste; and, as they consider this as the summum bonum of all good eating, so they figuratively call everything they think elegant and uncommon Macaroni . . . ") The Macaroni would set Great Britain's gender norms on fire. Who knew that a face full of foundation, a head full of powder, and living one's best life could cause such a delicious stir?

The Macaroni trend can be first traced to shortly after the Seven Years' War (1756–1763). With the war over, a travel ban was lifted, which allowed young, wealthy men to remedy their cabin fever and escape Great Britain. These youth would flock around the European continent in hordes for up to a year at a time in what was called the Grand Tour (you can think about it as a gap year of sorts), often ending their sojourns in Italy and France. There, they soaked up all the pop culture and fashion trends they'd been deprived of during the war. At the time, Paris and Southern Italy were the chicest destinations, where high-end fashion and beauty trends began. While there, these young people delighted in foreign sensibilities, excitedly adopting French styles of beauty with large wigs and ornate makeup, along with Italian sartorial trends: tighter silhouettes, more ostentatious accessories, and colors.

When they came back home, they brought a fresh aesthetic and perspective on life. At the time, English male attire was composed of baggier fits and monochromatic colors, with makeup-free complexions. Wigs were worn but had remained the traditional "scratch-wigs," which were modest, made with human and animal hair, in other words for dads and dads alone. To the youth, these wigs were worn only by dads and olds. Instead of blending into the monochromatic crowd, these men began walking—and *working*—the cobblestone streets of London in sparkling narrow heels, flashy outfits, and "feminine" makeup: stark-white foundation, rouged lips, and blushed cheeks. To top it off, these boys sported larger-than-life powdered wigs that towered over a couple of feet and were accessorized by beautiful tiny hats that sat on top like vibrant birds looking over their castlelike nests. These were *French* wigs that were *bon chic bon genre*—swaggy, cool, chic—inspired by *the* fashion idol himself, the late King Louis XIV. Highly perfumed, these wigs used globs of pomade to keep the hair in place, and tons of white powder to get it to French-level elegance. Tall in the front and thick in width, the fashionable wigs of this period ended in a long, thin tail at the back, "looking rather like a horse." To keep the pounds of product in their wigs from staining the backs of their extravagant jackets, these men started wearing wig-bags (literal bags that the wig tails could be stuffed into) as accessories. Their trendsetting ways soon began trickling into the suburbs, to rural towns, and out to the countryside. Soon enough, young men from the working, servant, and artisan classes were rocking Macaroni-style out and about. A popular cartoon called "What, is this my son Tom?," describes the phenomenon from a father's perspective. In it, a farmer, confused by his son's new sense of dress, pokes at the small hat sitting high on his massive wig with a cane, curious (and petrified) that Tom has adopted such a grotesque sense of dress. "The honest Farmer, come to Town, Can scarce believe his Son his own . . ." the caption reads.

It didn't stop and end at the wigs. Macaroni were obsessed with beauty and, just like any of the chicest women, used a variety of products to achieve that perfect porcelain look. Their powdered wigs matched their faces. There were antifreckle night masks, cold creams, tooth powders and breath-fresheners. Some were prescribed by physicians, others were home-made. Rouge would be placed triangularly on the middle of the lips in addition to getting blended into cheeks to create a sun-kissed, youthful radiance. Another popular beauty trend adopted by both men and women were beauty patches—these were velvet stickers cut in a shape such as a crescent moon, heart, diamonds, stars, or dot and used to hide pock marks.

And all of this was unsightly to older men, who thought it was improper and inappropriate for men to present themselves in such a flamboyant manner. The Macaroni were perceived by the older generations as being pretentious and excessive. The media quickly became obsessed with these young men, with magazines, journals, and reporters dedicated to documenting the Macaroni and their growing influence. One wrote that the "extravagant size of the macaroni's hairstyle seemed to speak at once to his embrace of artifice, deca-dence, and the pursuit of pleasure." Another published that "Such a figure, essenced and perfumed, with a bunch of lace sticking out under its chin, puzzles the common passenger to determine the *thing's* sex."

As dehumanizing and homophobic as that passage seems now, such language became the norm when it came to describing the Macaroni and their new dominance in British culture. It also shows just how threatened the older generation was when it came to a more liberal-minded and expressive future. The Macaroni would inspire paintings, sculptures, and plays. A series of portraits of Macaroni by husband-and-wife duo Matthew and Mary Darly would become world famous. The sketched pieces documented various Macaroni in their everyday lives on a plain background. Today, many of them are housed at the Metropolitan Museum of Art in New York City. The Macaroni would even inspire pop songs of the day like "Yankee Doodle." "Yankee Doodle went to town / Riding on a pony / Stuck a feather in his cap / And called it Macaroni" is a pop culture swipe at the "Yankee" Americans who were considered both clueless and uncultured. (Of course, Americans would later adopt the song and own the fact that they weren't as hoity-toity as the British . . .)

Such style and confidence—not to mention painstaking attention to detail—made these young Macaroni into dazzling, walking, talking pieces of artwork. While the Macaroni had an immense following when they first emerged on the scene, only a decade later, they'd find themselves out of favor. By the 1780s, they'd lose public opinion altogether after a decade of successful media campaigns launched against them. The many parody plays and songs written about them were no longer funny or perceived as innocent humor. The vitriolic messaging—which called them "effeminate," "women," "monkeys," "things," "homosex-ual," and even "hermaphrodites"—would again become despised. When the 1800s came, it was deemed taboo for men to wear makeup, wear fabulous clothing, and be so minutely interested in self-expression. The rise of the Enlightenment period inspired a new breed of intellectuals who perceived fashion and beauty as excess. This would usher in arguably the most boring period of expression, known as the Victorian era, where all semblance of vibrant fun was painted morose and somber black and white.

While the Macaroni endured extreme homophobia, bullying, and, later, rejection by their own people, their brief time at the forefront of culture forced rigid thinkers to reckon with different methods of masculine expression. Forced to fight for the space to simply exist, the Macaroni ultimately illuminate how young people have always strained against binaries . . . and how a little powder here and some lipstick there can do the world some good!

MACARONI BEAUTY MUST-HAVES

These beauty boys risked their lives for a perfect porcelain look. Their coveted beauty products held lethal doses of arsenic, lead, and mercury, which caused comas for the lucky ones and death for many others. Ironically, the more cosmetics they used, the worse their skin ended up looking. These cosmetics would cause eyes to swell, skin to inflame and blacken, teeth to decay, and hair to fall out.

Unfortunately, worsening complexions were great for cosmetic sales. After all, when one's face begins to melt away, beauty products to cover it become that much more essential. The following staples are in every typical Macaroni man's beauty bag.

Foundation: A DIY recipe instructed men to steep lead in a pot of vinegar and "rest it in a bed of manure for at least three weeks." The lead would soften, at which point, one should pound it into white powder.

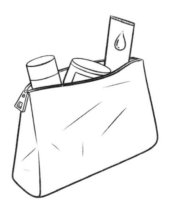

Powder: Made of flaky dried lead, powder was used from day to night to touch up one's complexion. (It was also used for wigs.)

Rouge: After the face was slathered with foundation and baked with lead flakes, these men applied pink rouge to their cheeks in a round or triangular shape. This gave a youthful, sun-kissed hint of color, adding dimension to their ghost-white complexions. At-home cosmetics recipe books like the popular *The Toilet of Flora* by Pierre-Joseph Buc'hoz gave tips on how to mix ceruse (a mixture of lead and vinegar), vermilion, arsenic, and mercury to create a long-lasting rouge paste.

Perfumed mouth water: It's said that the Macaroni would swish sweet-smelling water in their mouths as a sort of mouthwash. They also had breath mints to hide the stench of their rotting teeth—the toxic beauty products (creams and lotions) they used would attack the enamel.

Beauty patches: The best way to hide smallpox scars, cracking skin, or blemishes? Beauty patches. Made of black silk taffeta or velvet, the patches were shaped into round spots or beautiful shapes like a moon, heart, star, or diamond, and backed with a sticky adhesive. These artificial beauty marks could be placed on a cheek, above the eyebrows, or on the lips, to draw attention to certain areas of the face.

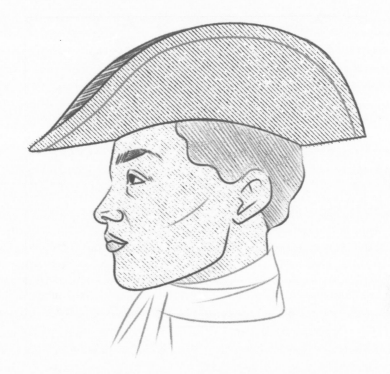

JULIUS SOUBISE

(1 7 5 4 - 1 7 9 8)

Meet Britain's Black Macaroni.

AT TEN YEARS OLD, JULIUS WAS PURCHASED AS A SLAVE IN the West Indies and taken to Great Britain by a captain named Stair Douglas. The captain eventually gave him as a gift to the Duchess of Queensberry, Catherine Hyde, who was smitten with the child. The duchess freed him, then adopted him, and, in spite of his displacement, raised him as her own—he was taught to fence, ride, and play the violin, and he grew into a charming tastemaker around town.

The young Julius was one of a handful of African British men who were able to make a place for themselves within British high society. It helped that rumors swirled around his origin story: it was said that he was a prince from Africa who had been captured, mistaken for a slave, before he was freed. As a young adult, Julius's predilections for beauty—ostentatious outfits, bright makeup, foppish wigs—allowed him to fit right in with other trendsetting Macaroni men. One could conjecture that like the other men, he, too, powdered his skin with white powders, which was en vogue at the time.

"He was expensive in perfume and wore nosegays," one journalist noted of his style and taste. His lone Black friend was a man named Ignatius Sancho, a writer and advocate who'd go on to make history as the first Black person to vote in a British general election. From Ignatius's journals, we get a glimpse of what life was like as a person of color at the time. He writes of the "national antipathy and prejudice" white British people had "towards their wooly headed brethren," and how, while he'd lived in Britain all his life, he'd never be accepted as British.

The media, who had been coming for the Macaroni already, would come for Julius in a particularly racist fashion. He was nicknamed "Mungo Macaroni"—the word "mungo" was a derogatory term for Black Brits that meant "servant." Soon, there were caricatures poking fun at his blackness and how peculiar it was that he ran in these aristocratic circles. One well-known painting depicts him fencing the duchess, his adopted mother who was still perceived by the public as his owner, while a bouquet of his signature nosegay flowers sits on the ground next to him.

Before Julius even made it to his thirties, he would be exiled to India by the duchess herself, after he was accused of attempting to rape of one of her maids. Horrified, she cut him off completely and forgot about him altogether. Julius would never see her or his fellow Macaroni friends ever again. Of course, nothing was proven one way or another, so we could also surmise that his very Blackness threatened the white household. And perhaps Julius became a Macaroni to tone down his own masculinity, and perceptions of threat to greater white Britain. Though we'll never know what truly occurred, we do know that at the end of his life, he had reinvented himself in Calcutta, and eventually set up a fencing school for boys and girls. In true Julius style, he knew how to not only survive, but thrive.

CLEANING UP

The stinking truth about bathing history.

THOUGH THE NOSE CAN DETECT MORE THAN 3 TRILLION UNIQUE scents, the irony is that you're unable to pick up on your own stench. Yes, we're looking at you, Europeans from the Middle Ages, ye who hath bathed twice a year. It has to do with the purpose of scent and how humans rely on the sense of smell for survival. Smell occurs when a molecule is collected onto receptors in your nose. The brain then picks up that information and hangs on to it, storing it away until it proves useful. With so many smells to process, including the work of discerning whether a certain scent is harmful or not, the brain doesn't tend to spare extra thought on anything that it comes into frequent contact with, and/or that seems relatively harmless. That's why, when you walk into a room and smell something unpleasant, your awareness of the odor usually fades away after a few minutes. If it's not going to kill you, your brain will get over it!

This explains how European societies could survive the funk of their collective body odor, best encapsulated in this quote from Saint Bernard of Clairvaux: "We all stink. No one smells." But unlike many European countries, not everyone around the world was accustomed to their body musk. From parts of Africa to Asia to precolonial North America, humans have been practicing the art of hygiene in their own unique ways throughout history. Some viewed bathing as a daily ritual for health, while others saw it as a religious practice.

Whether solo, communal, or in private spaces, in many ancient cultures, the act of bathing was closely attached to religion or some sort of higher power. The Egyptians or the ancient Babylonians saw cleansing as a purifying ritual. For Buddhists and Muslims, cleaning your body of impurities was also symbolic of clearing the mind and spirit. In Islam, followers must wash their bodies multiple times a day before praying.

For those who did choose to clean their bodies, a bath would entail dunking oneself in a natural water source: a river, lake, or ocean, or hot springs like the Vikings. Those without access to these natural sources of water had no choice but to create artificial spaces of water. The oldest example of this is the Great Bath of Mohenjo-daro, a public bathhouse in Pakistan. The massive tub, which was around 40 feet by 22 feet, can be traced back to 3000 BCE. There were two stairways that led into the bath from opposite ends. The sophisticated structure was watertight, with flooring made of finely fitted bricks plastered with mud. There was even a small hole used as a drain for dirty water.

Other sophisticated bathing structures, similar to what we'd now call showers, were pioneered by the Greeks. They installed these private bathing rooms in their gyms, where men went to train in public sports. *Gymnos* actually means "naked" in Greek, and men would go to the bathing rooms to wash off and hang out with other guys after their hard workouts. The Roman Empire would take bathing culture a bit further, dedicating an entire city as a spa: the city that is now Bath, England, was originally created as a getaway for Roman self-care enthusiasts who wanted to pamper themselves on the daily. Called Aquae Sulis, "the waters of Sul," after Sulis, the Celtic goddess of healing and sacred waters, and Minerva, the Roman goddess of wisdom, the city constructed multiple structures for large pools, in addition to structures for hot, warm, and cold bathtubs.

> Some viewed bathing as a daily ritual for health, while others saw it as a religious practice.

The fall of the Roman Empire in late 300s BCE led to Europe phasing out bathing altogether. Christians during the Middle Ages were hygiene rebels of sorts—to them, bathing became connected to sin. Christian doctrine promoted the idea that caring too much about your physical body was vain. That, and the fact that having to bathe is hardly mentioned in the Bible. If God didn't care, the thinking went, why should we? Many of the Roman bathing structures and plumbing systems in the city of Bath went out of use. Public bathhouses became perceived as unsanitary places, with the religious set viewing them much as they viewed brothels. There was stigma attached to visiting communal pools, as it was considered inappropriate to watch others in the nude.

It didn't help that Europe was plagued with pandemics, which led many to believe that bathing caused the pores to open up, making the body vulnerable to bacteria and disease. It's noted that even royals feared bathing. Queen Elizabeth I was said to have bathed once every three months—and that was considered excessive. Queen Isabella of Castile allegedly bathed twice in her life—once when she was born, and once before her wedding day. It's also noted that King Louis XIV bathed thrice in his life and had such bad breath that one of his mistresses allegedly doused herself in perfume so she wouldn't have to smell him.

While the Europeans became deathly afraid of washing their bodies, Asians—including the Japanese, Koreans, and Indians—had made it part of their daily lives. Bathing culture can be traced to Buddhist temples in India, where religious leaders cleansed themselves of evil thoughts and speech and elevated their minds as they washed their bodies. Followers of Buddha even celebrate his birthday by using fragrant water. As Buddhism spread into East Asia, China, Japan, and Korea created their own bathing rituals. The Japanese opened bathhouses, known as *onsen*, in the Edo Period, which lasted from the seventeenth through nineteenth centuries. Thousands were built on the natural hot springs scattered around the many islands of the country. Koreans had mogyoktang, kiln saunas that were used not only for hygiene, but for medicinal purposes as well. These saunas, run by Buddhist monks, who maintained the brick-lined bathhouses, were the precursors to today's modern Korean spas, which we know and love.

Bathing was a new phenomenon when it came to the United States. It was only in the mid-1800s that bathing culture became normalized. Though the modern shower had been invented in England a century before, it wouldn't be adopted by Americans until the Civil War. In 1861, at the start of the war, the US Sanitary Commission pioneered a new era of sanitation in order to help wounded soldiers in need of relief. Most of these soldiers healed simply by being hyperaware of their personal cleaning habits, and soon enough, the correlation between cleanliness and health had been instilled in all American households. Houses were equipped with their own rooms for bathing, and Americans adopted what would become our present habits for washing our hands, hair, bodies, and teeth.

> *The Dish Behind Soap: Soap works by trapping dirt and destroying viruses and bacteria in bubbles known as micelles, which wash away with water. One of the earliest recipes for soap dates from 2200 BCE—archaeologists uncovered a clay tablet from Babylon that detailed how to make a soap with evergreen tree oil, salt, and water.*

Today, the developed world perceives bathing as it does eating or sleeping: as a necessary part of one's day. It's also become a ritual to some, a luxury to others, and to still others remains a privilege. With Korean, Japanese, Russian, and Turkish spas having a resurgence of popularity in cities around the globe, newer generations are discovering the art of the bath. And there are constant new innovations pushing enthusiasm for cleanliness forward, from waterless shampoos to CBD bath salts to vegan body washes and more. It's a good time to be alive and putting your best smell, and hygiene, forward! After all, your nose really is judging you.

According to some reports, Queen Elizabeth I fell victim to her beauty products. At the time, the most popular cosmetic was "Venetian ceruse," a mixture of white lead and vinegar that was used to cover pockmarks. In turn, it slowly killed its users as the lead seeped into their bloodstream, poisoning them to death. Some accounts report that Elizabeth's coffin exploded because of the noxious vapors emanating from her rotting corpse.

Thankfully, in our modern age, we've cut out most, if not all, traces of arsenic, mercury, and lead in cosmetics. At this point, the European Union has identified and banned over a thousand hazardous chemicals found in personal care products. Meanwhile, in the US? Only eleven. It's one reason why celebrities to beauty influencers have pushed for "clean beauty" (a term popularized by the Queen of Goop, Gwyneth Paltrow). While the actress has come under fire for "greenwashing," the American beauty industry's rules haven't been updated for more than a century, meaning there are few safety regulations. In fact, the FDA has no authority to even recall unsafe beauty products; it's up to the manufacturer of the tainted product to do so itself.

Consumers are trying to keep brands accountable and transparent in their ingredient listing, but the term "clean beauty" is far from defined. Ask any expert and they'll give you a different answer. And retailers from Sephora and Ulta to clean beauty–focused Credo all have their own definitions of which ingredients are "clean." So where does one even start?

Read Your Ingredients: Though there are plenty of disagreements when it comes to what's considered toxic, there are some ingredients that most (if not all) agree are unsafe. These include parabens (a preservative linked with breast cancer); mineral oils (fillers like petroleum, paraffinum liquidum or liquid paraffin, petrolatum); sodium lauryl sulfate (SLS, a product that removes oils); aluminum compounds (found in antiperspirants); talc (powders linked to cancer); oxybenzone (a chemical found in sunscreens that can harm the coral reefs); fragrances (over 1 percent in the ingredient list means that brands can hide the exact ingredients included); ethoxylated oxide (known to be a carcinogen); formaldehyde (a compound found mostly in shampoos—and used to embalm corpses!— that can cause severe reactions); hydroquinone (a skin lightener linked to cancer and organ function failure); triclosan (an antibacterial agent linked with decreased thyroid hormone production); and silica (a thickening agent linked to cancer).

Know Your Buzzwords: Clean? Green? Vegan? What are all these marketing terms? Here's a quick breakdown . . .

- *Nontoxic*—This most likely means that a beauty product includes no ingredients found on the EU's more stringent list of banned substances. American brands that use "nontoxic" are signaling that they've eliminated any and all of these ingredient no-nos.
- *Vegan*—The term "vegan" means the product includes no ingredients derived from animals or animal by-products, including honey. But just because it's vegan doesn't mean it's necessarily nontoxic. A brand can use only vegan ingredients but still contain (vegan) toxic chemical ingredients.
- *Sustainable or Green*—This means there is no by-product that does harm to the planet. (This does not exclude the product from potentially doing harm to your body.) From the packaging to the chemicals in the formula to the ethically sourced ingredients (meaning not obtained from endangered plants or animals)— "sustainable" is a difficult classification for any beauty brand to achieve, especially since most beauty packaging is still not

100 percent recyclable. But the industry is getting there, and fast, with an increase in PCR (post-consumer resin) usage, among other types of recycled plastics.

- *Organic*—In order for a product to be labeled "organic," a classification regulated by the USDA, any ingredient in the product needs to be at least 95 percent organic. This means that there are no genetically modified ingredients or pesticides. But just because a product is organic doesn't mean it's necessarily more effective, or safer. Also keep in mind that smaller indie brands can't afford USDA organic certification because of how expensive it is. This means a brand can technically be organic, but without the funds to pay for the certification, couldn't market their products as such.

- *Cruelty-Free*—This means the product has not been tested on animals. Yes, there are still some brands that test cosmetics on rabbits in places in the world. But times they are a-changin'! Recently, China announced it would end the cruel practice. It's less common in the US, where more consumers have demanded bans on animal testing in the cosmetics industry.

So What *Is* Clean? In general, "clean" means nontoxic, environmentally conscious, plant-based, and good for you *and* the planet. But it's a vague term that means different things to different people, and ultimately, you'll have to make your own decisions on what "clean" means to you. A product might be vegan, environmentally friendly, *and* nontoxic, but still use packaging that isn't sustainable. That may be okay for some people, but a deal-breaker for others. Additionally, synthetic ingredients aren't always your enemy. Many synthetics are not only nontoxic but also work toward making your product more stable and effective. Always keep in mind that "clean" is also a marketing term used by brands to sell you their goods. Be vigilant, be aware, and stay informed.

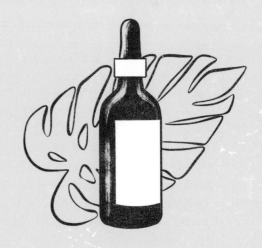

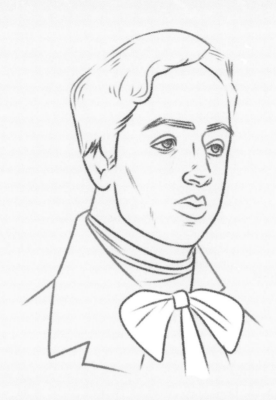

BEAU BRUMMELL

(1 7 7 8 - 1 8 4 0)

Five grooming rules from the 1700s.

THERE'S EAU DE TOILETTE. THEN THERE'S EAU DE *TOILET*.

Thankfully, the smelly state of British hygiene would finally change with the arrival of a certain influencer who'd make baths cool again. Beau Brummell would not only become Britain's best-known fashionista, ushering in a more modest sense of style called dandyism, but also its grooming savior. He was the anti-Macaroni in every sense, doing away with any makeup, cosmetics, and colorful embellishments. Brummell's influence was only amplified through his BFF, King George IV, who would take cues from him. Soon the grooming revolution would change British culture for the better.

Below, Beau Brummell's grooming rules to live by:

1. **Wash thy body like thy clothes.** Men during this time period were so serious about keeping their clothes clean that they'd hang them to dry in the fields of Islington. This, so they'd have a country smell to them, but also to avoid the soot from the city's many factories. Brummell brought up a good point to many naysayers who questioned his grooming advice: If one's clothes were to be cleaned, so should the body underneath it all. After all, if the body is drenched with dirt, the bright white shirts would become discolored as well.

2. **Thou shalt refrain from perfume.** At the time, refraining from a fragrance like a rich cologne was like not wearing deodorant—without it, you must live on the fringes of culture, bound to be sniffed at and judged. But Brummell had a great point. Instead of masking body odor with the scents popular at the time (geranium, musk, and civet, among others), people should try to prevent stenches by bathing instead. A revolutionary concept, really!

3. **The "chafe" is not safe.** In the nineteenth century, most people did something called "chafing": instead of cleansing the body with water, one would take a wool or cambric towel and vigorously rub it against the skin. Perspiration was thought to help maintain optimal health and rid the body of toxins. To chafe was to wipe down the body without stripping it of its natural sweat and grime, but Brummell introduced the idea that soaking in hot water was a lot more effective at protecting oneself from disease.

4. **Thou shalt bathe like no tomorrow.** Until the 1800s, most households lacked private bathing facilities, so people frequented public bathhouses instead, which were far from the most hygienic places. Knowing this, the germophobic Brummell had his own private bath in his home, an obvious luxury. He'd heat up gallons of water and pour it into his tub, where he'd soak for hours on end. Some record him as bathing for up to four hours. The professional socialite, whose lifestyle was supported entirely by his wealthy friends, took his sweet time, to the point that many of those friends would come over for meetings and conversations while he soaked. Apparently, he "kept the door to his bedroom ajar so that he could carry on a conversation while he washed, shaved, and dressed."

5. **Equip thyself.** What did every man need in his bathroom? According to Brummell, milk, which has natural exfoliative properties from its lactic acid (to soften skin); a coarse body brush for exfoliating; shaving soap cakes; brushes made of badger hair (for facial hair maintenance); razors; nail brushes; tweezers for "stray hairs"; and, of course, a dentist's magnifying mirror. He also kept his breath fresh all day and was one of the first to keep up a daily toothbrushing regimen, one that would influence his many peers in Britain's upper echelon. This new code of modesty and cleanliness would impact generations to come.

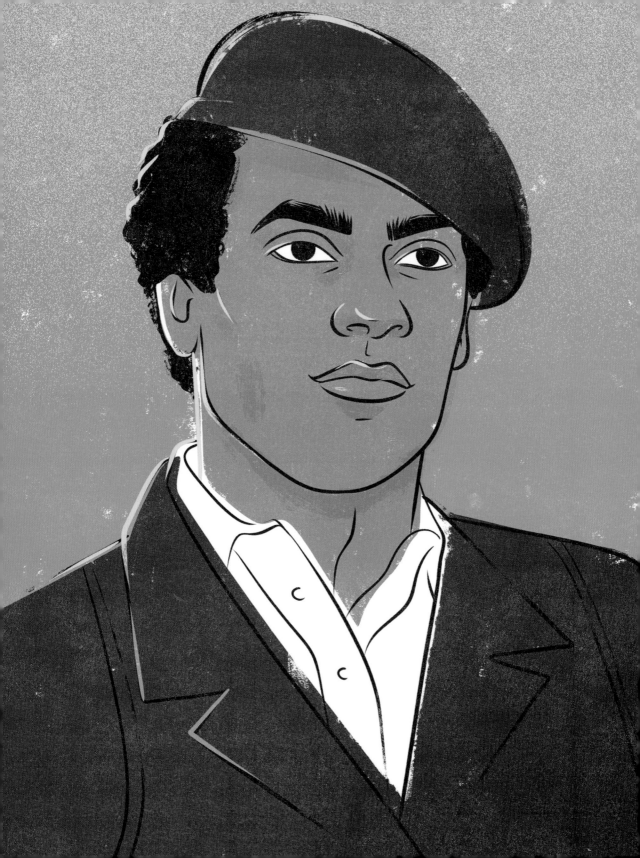

BLACK PANTHER PARTY

(1966–1982)

And the politics of hair.

AFTER CENTURIES OF COLONIZATION, ENSLAVEMENT, OPPRESSION, and an international emphasis on whiteness, the Black Panther Party, a grassroots militant organization that emerged in the 1960s to reclaim Black power, heritage, and identity, would finally begin to shift the dominant cultural narrative around beauty. "The reason for it, you might say," said Black Panther Kathleen Cleaver in 1968, "is like a new awareness among black people that their own natural physical appearance is beautiful and is pleasing to them." For Huey P. Newton, socialist activist and cofounder of the party, hair was a means of fighting for change—hair could unite young people in a singular fashion, and show the world what it looked like be uncompromisingly Black. Newton was someone who fought against the government by using his head—and hair—first.

As a child, Newton noticed that no one grew out their natural hair. Not the women who sat in the pews of his father's Baptist church. Not the men who congregated at local barbershops.

Not even rock stars like Little Richard (see page 187 for more on Little Richard) or James Brown, who wore theirs "conked," or straightened. It bothered him that everyone he looked up to had been taught to be ashamed of who they were, still tethered to white culture and the desire for acceptance that had been enforced during enslavement.

From the beginning of America, black hair has been used as a means of suppression and oppression within African American communities. Before the abolition of slavery, enslaved Africans had their heads forcibly shaved as a means of stripping them of their cultural identity and dignity. After Congress passed the 13th Amendment, ending legal slavery in 1865, newly freed slaves were encouraged to integrate into society, at a cost: they had to adhere to white beauty norms. Many would straighten their hair with hot tools or harmful chemicals that would burn their scalps.

But the dialogue began to shift with Malcolm X and the inception of the civil rights movement. Hair relaxing is a process that involves an entire day of work. "I gritted my teeth and tried to pull the sides of the kitchen table together," Malcolm wrote in his memoir. "The comb felt as if it was raking my skin off. My eyes water, my nose was running. I couldn't stand it." His rejection of conking would spark a generation of young people to embrace their whole selves.

Huey Newton would go on to attend Merritt College in Oakland, California, where he befriended Bobby Seale, a future cofounder of the Black Panther Party. "I questioned what was happening in my own family and in the community around me," Newton noted of this time period in his memoir, *Revolutionary Suicide.* Unlike Martin Luther King Jr., whose peaceful protests were garnering support from middle-class white Americans, Newton began to realize the necessity of a militant method of demanding change. And unlike King, who cropped his hair short and wore button-down shirts and slacks, Newton grew his hair out and wore all black. The Black community could no longer be ashamed of who they were, he thought. More so, they couldn't afford to continue asking for permission on the political and cultural fronts from the greater white powers that be.

After the Black Panthers formed, thousands of young Americans quickly joined the cause. Young people everywhere were mobilizing through their local communities, protesting at statehouses, rallying in cities, and promoting Black love and positivity through the Black Is Beautiful movement. Members of the Black Panther Party proudly identified themselves with a distinct style of dress, making it easy to spot each other in a crowd—the iconic uniform included fitted leather jackets, sunglasses, berets, and ever-growing Afros.

For the Panthers, growing their hair out was self-love, and a middle finger to the government. More so, the growth of natural hair was symbolic of rejecting systemic suppression. "We had been completely brainwashed and we didn't even know it," Assata Shakur, a former

Black Liberation Army member—and the late Tupac Shakur's godmother—later said. "We accepted White value systems and White standards of beauty and, at the time, we accepted the White man's view of ourselves."

Black Panther members began using custom Afro picks with a raised fist on the handle, to not only style their hair, but as a physical reminder of their push toward change. Sometimes worn in the hair as an accessory, each comb came with a black fist molded at the end of the handle. It was an emblem of solidarity against respectability politics.

While there was a celebration of Afros, there remained fear in wearing them out. As a young black person, flaunting long natural hair made you an easy target for the police. In 1967, Newton was arrested on murder charges (but was later acquitted). And in 1968, Seale was arrested for his involvement in demonstrations that took place during the Democratic National Convention in Chicago. A couple of months later, two Panthers were killed by police, an order made by the FBI. In 1970, Angela Davis, a prominent Communist and Black Panther, became the third woman to be listed on the FBI's 10 Most Wanted Fugitives list. FBI director J. Edgar Hoover said the Panthers were "the greatest threat to internal security of the country." Older generations panicked, and tried convincing their children to cut it short—but as the tense standoffs went on, Afros remained.

The growth of natural hair was symbolic of rejecting systemic suppression.

The Black Panther Party would remain active for the next decade, and their aesthetics would begin inspiring pop culture. The movement inspired mainstream figures from the Jackson 5 to Jimi Hendrix to NBA player Julius Erving to grow their hair out. But as Afros became more accepted, the Black Panther Party was being forced apart.

Newton had fled to Cuba after being investigated for murder. When he returned from exile in 1977, the movement had changed; in the interim, many leaders had taken the party in multiple directions. The Panthers had split from within, with some members wanting to continue their struggle against the police, and others believing their time was better spent in public service and government cooperation. By 1980, there were only twenty-seven active members of the party. Newton lived a slightly quieter life, writing books and studying ideologies, until his murder by gunfire in 1989, by a member of the Black Guerrilla Family, a Black prison and street gang. The gang had been at war with Newton and the Black Panther Party for twenty years.

Though the Black Panther Party may be no more, their legacy and spirit live on. Afro hair persists as a powerful symbol of Blackness, pride, and style. From runways to magazines, pop culture and more, Afros remain a symbol of Black Power, though hair continues to be as political as ever. With continued discrimination against natural hair, a new generation of activists are calling for change. Recently, a law called the CROWN Act—an acronym for "Create a Respectful and Open World for Natural Hair"—was introduced in California to protect black and brown Americans from workplace or school discrimination stemming from their hair or the way they chose to wear it. Here's to the CROWN Act, the Black Panther Party's years of activism, and the continued fight for freedom of identity.

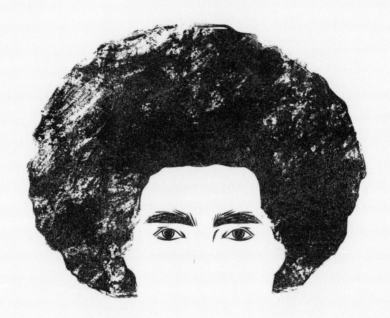

GROW YOUR BEST HAIR EVER,
INSPIRED BY THE AFRO MOVEMENT

Let it grow!

Whether you're growing your hair into an Afro or locs, or want simply stronger, healthier hair, we've rounded up the best hair tips from celebrity stylist Vernon Scott, who counts folks like Pharrell Williams, Kanye West, Idris Elba, Maxwell, and Jaden Smith, among others, as clients. Here Scott takes us through every product you need, how to use it, and the one secret for your best 'fro ever.

1. KEEP IT NATURAL.
Healthy hair starts with better products, says Scott. For beautifully grown-out hair, Scott suggests using non-synthetic ingredients. "The leaves on a tree are equally important as the soil that is growing from," he says. "Meaning, you need to give your scalp love as you do your hair." His favorites include essential oils like vitamin E, coconut, jojoba, and kukui nut oils. "Whole Foods or Trader Joe's have amazing organic coconut butters and oils—I swear by them." Then, since hair is made of keratin, you'll want to replenish and strengthen it with protein treatments, followed by deeply moisturizing conditioners. Major retailers and drugstores carry leave-in keratin or conditioning treatments.

2. WASH. CO-WASH. REPEAT.
"It's all about ensuring your hair has nutrients and isn't depleted of moisture," Scott says. He suggests washing with shampoo up to three times a month to avoid irritating the scalp. In between, Scott says to co-wash (that's washing with conditioner only) or just rinsing hair briefly after a workout or if you've been sweating.

3. JUST ADD MOISTURE.
"Anything that's moisturized will grow—think about a plant," says Scott. "The thing with our hair is that it's exposed to so many different things on a natural level and then on a manipulation level, so be gentle and replenish with a moisturizer. After you shower, dry and moisturize; most people forget to seal [moisture] in. This is perhaps something I can't stress enough." After washing and drying, seal moisture in with an organic coconut oil to encourage health and growth. "It seals the hair follicles and closes it so it becomes hydrated and smooth," he says.

PRO TIP: Try not to add intense heat to dry, says Scott. "It works against moisture retention and overall health of hair." Instead, towel dry and moisturize your hair while it still feels damp. "Your hair will soak in the moisturizer much better."

Cream- or water-based moisturizers on drugstore shelves are good, but essential oils are still best.

4. CHECK ON IT.
The easiest way to check if your hair is well on its way? Its shine factor. "If your hair is healthy, it will be radiant," says Scott. "It's like your skin. If you take care of it and you have a regimen, your hair will have this healthy glow." But on the flip side, if your hair isn't happy, it'll tell you. One obvious sign? "It becomes straight as a pin," he says. "That's because all of the essential oils and nutrients are stripped from it. It can also be from heat damage. There are so many factors. Long story short, be gentle, check in, and pamper yourself." Remember, hair care is a journey—there are no shortcuts, but it will be worth it.

Pretty

THE RITUALS AND
PRACTICES OF BEAUTY HAVE
ALWAYS BEEN SHARED
THROUGH COMMUNITY.

Fierce

FROM LEARNING TO FEEL BETTER IN YOUR own skin to celebrating important experiences within one's tribe, beauty has been a formative aspect of individual and collective identities. In this section, we uncover the individuals and groups who channel, or have created, beauty legacies. From nonbinary folx who have been vital to their respective collectives around the world to drag queens who strutted right into *herstory* to Black entrepreneurs who created the products their people needed—meet the fierce icons who made spaces for themselves, and in doing so, brought their communities closer together.

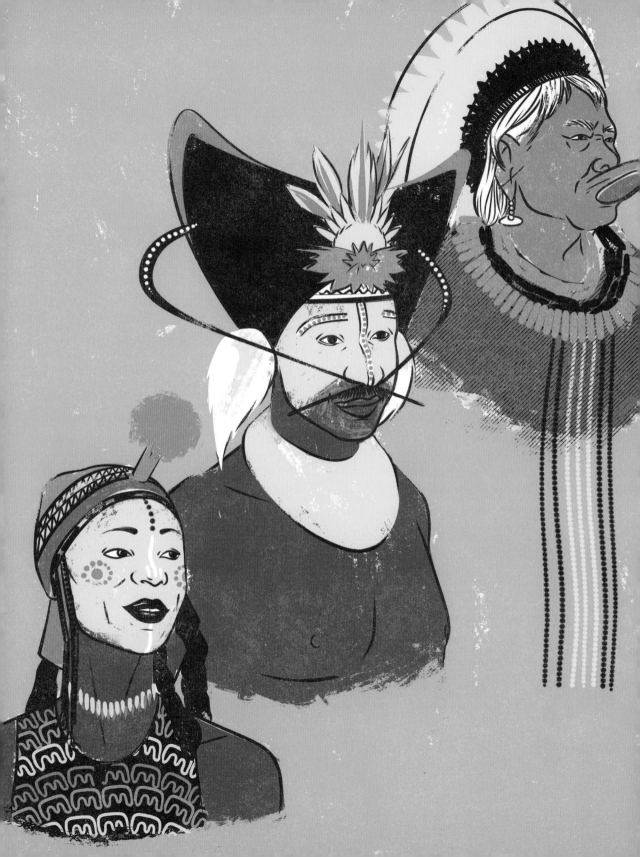

(PRETTY) BOYS TO MEN

Beauty rituals, pageantry, and magic throughout the world.

FOR MANY INDIGENOUS TRIBES AROUND THE WORLD, YOU MUST become beautiful before you become a man. To primp, pamper, and beautify your face, body, and hair is seen in many cultures as a sacred tradition.

THE HULI WIGMEN of Papua New Guinea

DEEP IN PAPUA NEW GUINEA'S SOUTHERN HIGHLANDS live the beautiful and ostentatious Huli tribe, known as "Wigmen" for the long, luscious wigs they take particular care in crafting from their own hair. The entire culture is centered around personal decoration and dress, with the men spending hours painting their faces and bodies on special occasions, growing out their hair, and creating elaborate headdresses from their hair and highly coveted ornaments like bird-of-paradise feathers. Wigs are essential to men. The bigger the hair, the more esteemed. As such, a man is able to flex his muscle through his ability to grow the healthiest and longest strands of hair to be created into elaborate wigs.

Unmarried men live with other bachelors, isolated from the rest of their community. During this time, they're guided by master Wigmen, who teach them spells, rituals, and the proper diets to help grow shiny, healthy hair. They'll spend the next few months (up to eighteen months) crafting their wigs. It's during this time that these young men are tasked at keeping their hair growth at an optimum. They are required to moisturize their hair three times a day, prohibited from sleeping in any manner that may squash their mane from growing, and asked not to eat spicy foods or fats, ingredients that are believed to inhibit locks from reaching their greatest potential. And then there are spells. Lots and lots of magic goes into these months in which sacred priests and elders will bless these young ones in the hopes of expanding their tresses. While all Huli men have more than one wig, the hair for those wigs must be grown and collected before a man is married. The results are incredible, statuesque, one-of-a-kind headdresses interspersed with flowers and feathers.

When the headdresses are complete, the Wigmen will paint their faces bright yellow, with red and white edges, using charcoal as a base coat, to transform themselves into "man-bird" hybrids. It's a sacred practice, as the charcoal paint comes from what the Huli call the "tree of the ancestors." Mixed with vegetable oils, the resulting thick pastes are also blended into facial hair and used as contour to sharpen features and pronounce the "beak." Noses are pierced with accessories like mother-of-pearl, bone, or feathers. To complete the look, men will wrap snakeskin around their heads and don beaded necklaces. And like the birds of paradise whose feathers adorn their headdresses, Huli women have far less colorful and elaborate styles.

THE KAYAPÓ of Brazil

BRAZIL'S INDIGENOUS PEOPLE HAVE RECEIVED INTERNATIONAL attention due to their protests against government encroachment on their land. In particular, images of the Kayapó marching in Brazilian streets against deforestation and mercury pollution, demanding to be seen and heard, drew the media's eye. The Kayapó refused to assimilate to a Western style of dress, choosing instead to march in their native attire—body paint, lip plates, headdresses, and all.

Before the Kayapó were forced into the public eye to protect their Amazonian territories, scrutinized by the media, and made the poster people for indigenous activists, they were a peaceful tribe who adhered to long-held traditions and rituals virtually untouched by colonizers. The Kayapós' entire lives center around a sacred rite where they become *mereremex*, which translates to "people who extend their beauty." It's a rite of passage for men before marriage, a process that includes adorning their bodies with accessories from head-to-toe, in addition to body modifications like lip plates. Lip plates are specific to men, and reach larger sizes depending on age. Boys are pierced shortly after birth, using a string of beads or mussel shells to keep the piercing from closing. Plugs range from cylindrical wood, to slick rock crystal.

But mereremex is spiritual as well—painting their skin in a multitude of colors allows other tribe members to "read" the symbols and decode each members' lineage, family history, and ancestry. The body paint comes in two colors: black and red, and unique symbols are given to each tribe member in the forms of lines and dots. Black paint is applied to specific areas of the body that are thought of as natural sources of energy. These are the upper arms, thighs, trunk, and internal and reproductive organs. Red is associated with vitality, energy, and a person's personal qualities. Usually painted on the eyes and mouth, they are symbolic of ideas, dreams, and speech. The symbols on the tribes members' bodies also allow shamans to conjure spirits and speak to them through song.

Each photograph of the Kayapó marching, with their faces painted in black and red, headdresses, and lip plates, capture not just an individual but an entire lineage fighting to save what is most important to them.

THE WODAABE of Niger

IMAGINE TINDER WHERE YOU FLAUNT YOUR GOODS IN PERSON to be swiped on IRL. For the nomadic Wodaabe tribe, men must compete in an annual beauty pageant in which the women are the judges and have complete control. And winners take what that they can get, whether that's a partner, a friends with benefits, or a position as upgraded spouse.

The annual weeklong festival, held in September, is called Gerewol, and migrating groups throughout the region trek across the semiarid steppes of the Sahel for a reunion. For Gerewol, the men go all out, beautifying for six hours a day, using ostrich feathers and poms made of yarn to make themselves seem taller. They paint their faces red with ochre; line their noses with black, white, and yellow patterns to emphasize their size; and apply black eyeliner and lipstick. Eyebrows are shaped into perfect swoops, and shells braided into their hair to symbolize wealth and fertility jangle on their bare chests as they dance to different beats. The pageantry also includes singing, and the baring of white teeth, a sign of masculinity and good health. The grand prize? Finding a new lover if you're tired of the old, even if you're both already married. "I've already spotted three men here that I like," the BBC quoted a married Wodaabe woman saying. "Stealing wives is not an easy thing," a Wodaabe tribesman once told *National Geographic*. Apparently, he's been chosen by thirty wives in his entire life, thanks to his hard work.

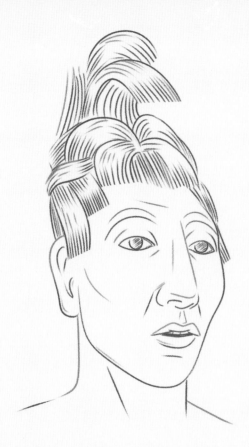

K'INICH JANAAB' PAKAL

(603–683 CE)

When your features pop.

"YOU'RE SO SEXY, YOU LOOK LIKE CORN."

An ear-catching pickup line in today's day for sure, but if you were an ancient Mayan, it may have been music to yours. Bad puns aside, Mayans viewed corn as the ultimate symbol of desirability. Maize (aka corn) was at the center of every Mayan's life—it was a sacred plant that was crucial to survival. Mayans had worshipped Yum Kaax, the god of maize. And according to their doctrine, corn birthed human beings, so the closer one resembled the plant—having an elongated head, hair styled like husk, and kernel-shaped teeth—the more attractive they were thought to be. "[Mayans] invested vast wealth and endured unspeakable pain to make themselves beautiful," confirms one professor. And the epitome of Mayan beauty had to be ruler K'inich Janaab' Pakal—by the end of his life, the influential man had achieved the utmost in physicality in every sense and set the standards for beauty during his time.

When K'inich was born in what is the current state of Chiapas, Mexico, Mayan parents would place two wooden boards alongside a newborn's head on both sides, squeezing the softness so the baby's forehead sloped forward and its head grew upward. The painstaking result was a divine corn-shaped skull that peaked toward the sky. K'inich's parents also tied a ball to his hair to dangle between his eyes, hoping he would be permanently cross-eyed, another signifier of attractiveness at the time. This was to resemble Kinich Ahau, the cross-eyed sun god, who also had an aquiline jaw. As he ascended to the throne at the age of twelve, he pierced his ears, lips, nose, and more—precious jewelry, in particular jade and other green stones, hung around his body. Body paint and tattoos were essential as well, in addition to scarification for select men.

Perhaps more important than accessories and tattoos were modified and embellished teeth. The procedure was only accessible for the wealthy, and it wasn't just expensive—it was excruciating as well. K'inich went through multiple rounds of dental procedures to have his teeth filed into T-shapes, signifying that he was a spiritual deity, and shaved down to resemble kernels. Teeth were also rearranged into decorative zigzag and blinged out. Long before grills became a modern trend, the Mayans embedded precious stones, including pyrite, hematite, turquoise, and jade, into their incisors. (Fun fact: Up to three stones could fit into a single tooth.) K'inich also used a prosthetic nose piece made from clay or plaster to enhance its already curved silhouette. It was placed on his nasal bridge to make it appear more beaklike. And to top off his beautiful, corn-esque look, K'inich grew out his hair into a long, shaggy bob that grazed his shoulders and was styled so it swooped over his forehead, the silky strands dangling above his brows like husks.

When he died in 683 CE, K'inich had ruled the Maya for over sixty-eight years, longer than any other ruler in the Americas. The beloved, intricately beautified man was buried in a temple inside a custom-made sarcophagus with incredibly detailed etching on its exterior. Considered a global treasure for its rich symbols, iconography, and design, much of the sarcophagus remains indecipherable. But the message in the care that went into its crafting is crystal clear: this ruler was perceived as nothing less than exceptional.

When's the last time you got a nice brow job?

Eyebrows, aka Upper Eyeball Fur, are the oft-forgotten brothers of the face. "They're part of your personality if you like it or not," says Joseph Carrillo, makeup artist and groomer to stars like Paris Hilton, Alexa Chung, and Taylor Schilling. "People will notice them for better or for worse. Eyebrows are your face's accessories; they enhance what you have. They can frame your dreamy eyes."

According to Joseph, current eyebrow trends range from the clean and defined look (think any and all K-pop stars) to more natural and fuller brows, à la Zayn Malik. But don't get it twisted, Joseph says. Bigger and hairier brows do not warrant allowing the hair to grow like wild weeds. For those who don't have naturally thick brows, you can work with what you have like Nick Jonas, or thicken them (read on for an easy hack).

For most men, plucking with tweezers is the best way of grooming the brows. Others can try waxing or threading for more noticeably shaped brows, though you can also try to find an expert who knows how to do them in a subtle, less sculpted way.

But you too can do your own brows—we swear, it's so plucking easy!

WHAT YOU'LL NEED:
- Tweezers
- Mirror
- Something long and straight (a comb or a brush is great)
- Brow gel or tinted eye gel

Show restraint. Remember these words, my friend: Do not overpluck. Do not overtweeze. Less is more. If your perfectionist tendencies kick in and you start tweezing away, you might end up eyebrow bald. For most guys, simply plucking *gently* does the trick.

Follow the rule of fourths. There's a rule of fourths when it comes to plucking your brows. If you're looking to find the perfect areas to pluck, take a look at the graphic below.

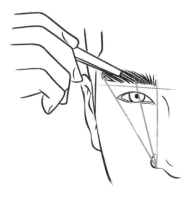

- Starting with the inner brow, place a brush or comb or anything straight on your face, trying to create a line from your inner eyebrow to your outer nostril. Pluck anything outside that line, and repeat on the other side.
- Align the brush or comb from your iris (that's the center of your eye) diagonally upward to your eyebrow. When it hits, you know that's your arch—pluck anything above that.
- Finally, align the brush or comb from the outside of your eye upward to your eyebrow. That's where your eyebrow should end. Pluck anything outside that line. Again, try not to overpluck.
- Get your brush or comb and lay it straight below you brows, just a little above the eyes. This is where your hairs should stop. Pluck any strays.
- Finish with your brow gel (any will do). A gel comb will simply style the gel in the right direction. If you want heavier brows, get a tinted gel for more beautiful, bushier eyebrows. Whatever you're using, comb your brows upward, then outward, with the brush.

BEYOND THE BINARY

Third genders around the world.

A FLUID FUTURE IS UPON US! WHILE THERE'S NO DOUBT THAT younger people are leading the charge when it comes to the gender revolution, the idea of a gender expression and identity outside the binary is not new. Gender nonconforming people have existed throughout time and throughout the world. Long before the rise of "they/them" pronouns in Western culture, nonbinary individuals, in some cultures dubbed "third gender," held a revered space among their respective peoples (though many now face frequent discrimination and lack of legal rights and recognition). These include the hijras of India, the khawaja sira of Pakistan, Two-Spirit people from many Indigenous tribes in North America, muxes from Mexico, mahu from Hawaii, the fa'afafine of Polynesia, among others.

Many third gender people were perceived as a vital part of their communities. Indian hijras have long held important positions in courts and administrations, in particular during the sixteenth through nineteenth centuries. Respected as religious leaders, they are sought out for blessing ceremonies and invited to attend special gatherings. The British attempted to erase hijras from Indian culture, stating that these "eunuchs" were "ungovernable" people of "filth, disease, contagions and contamination" and a "threat to colonial political authority." But hijras continued to fight for freedom against oppressive colonial rule. Today, hijras are recognized by the Indian government as a third gender and can express themselves through makeup, piercings, and femme-presenting clothing, though they are sadly not as respected as they were several centuries ago—many now rely on sex work, and face discrimination, abuse, and violence.

In Oaxaca, Mexico, a third gender known as muxes live in a small region called Istmo de Tehuantepec. According to legend, the muxe came into being after a saint named Vicente Ferrer came into town spreading different seeds: male, female, and a mixed bag. The result from the latter were the muxes.

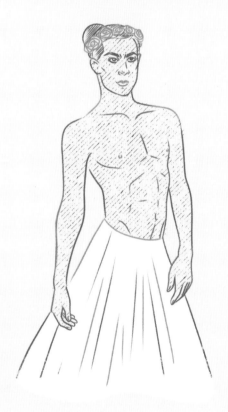

Since precolonial Spain, the muxes have blurred the lines between traditional masculinity and femininity, expressing themselves with vibrant makeup, colorful clothing, and beautiful accessories. It makes it simpler linguistically that the Zapotec language spoken in the region does not use gender-specific pronouns. Oaxaca is considered somewhat of a "queer paradise"—there, it is culturally accepted for muxe to date, marry, and carry on romances with women or men, neither party labeled as being LGBTQIA.

In Hawaii individuals known as mahu were considered sacred beings who expressed themselves with both the divine feminine and divine masculine. They played an essential role in teaching their communities about the balance of masculinity and femininity throughout an individual's lifespan. Considered a third gender, the mahu were respected priests and historians, who passed down generational stories. The keepers of cultural traditions and ceremonies, they were essential in sharing historic knowledge to future generations. Many parents would ask a mahu to name their children, "for mixed-gender individuals are recognized as special, compassionate, and creative," said one historian. Today, those who value the mahu consider them healers and teachers who maintain native Hawaiian traditions. But not all mahu have been shown love. There are still many who are rejected due to the remnants of colonization and rampant anti-LGBTQIA sentiment in Hawaii.

In Polynesia, the very word *fa'afafine* literally translates to "in the manner of woman." Said to have the "fa'afafine spirit," these individuals are celebrated as being able to navigate two genders. As such, these third-gendered individuals take on more duties of a Samoan woman, including responsibilities within their households. Today, Polynesian culture is socially conservative, and is heavily influenced by Christianity—it's still not acceptable for a man to cross-dress or express himself through traditionally feminine clothing or makeup. However, the fa'afafine, as a third gender, can live outside those confines, and choose to take up relationships with other men or with women. Though there are now only around five hundred fa'afafine in Samoa, they're beloved by their people, and frequently have roles as caretakers within their communities.

Probably the most recognized third gender people are from Thailand. Called *kathoey*, they have been vital members of Thai society for hundreds of years. Thailand, a predominantly Buddhist country, has had much more of an embrace of fluid gender identity compared to other Asian countries, perhaps because it is one of the only in that region to have remained relatively free from Western colonial influence. Thailand considers a gender system based on three genders, according to Richard Totman, a professor and author of *The Third Sex: Kathoey—Thailand's Ladyboys.*

In modern Thailand, kathoey have become synonymous with trans women assigned male at birth, or those who consider themselves a third gender, altogether. Fully integrated into culture, the kathoey are represented in a variety of industries, and are known for their beauty. With their faces full of the best cosmetic techniques and their lush hair, many have gone on to become national celebrities. But in spite of how normalized they are in Thailand, the country has failed to protect everyday kathoey citizens from being exploited by Westerners for entertainment or sex, so much so that it's said that the 200,000 sex workers produce up to $4.5 billion GDP a year, roughly 1 percent of Thailand's entire economy. Their popularity in the West has also come with insulting names like "ladyboys," a pejorative that refuses to acknowledge their real identities. While kathoey may be known internationally in association with the Thai nightlife industry, they are represented much more widely in Thai culture—some, like Parinya Charoenphol, are Muy Thai champions; Treechada Petcharat is one of many actresses and social media stars who has millions of followers; and Tanwarin Sukkhapisit, the first kathoey politician, can currently be seen representing Thailand's Future Forward Party.

Whether adding zest to *E! News* fashion commentary, dancing alongside Taylor Swift in her pastel-hued "You Need to Calm Down" music video, or dazzling as a host for a viral K-pop drag show, Chester Lockhart ebbs and flows into any role in Hollywood with ease. Here's how Chester went from an awkward Las Vegas teen to a fierce, inspirational, otherworldly multihyphenate who continues to pave the way forward for themselves on their own terms.

....

I definitely had a difficult time accepting myself while growing up in an ultraconservative white-trash town. My parents are devout Christians and were super active in the church when I was growing up. I felt really isolated as I became more aware of my otherness as a teenager and struggled immensely to fit in at school.

As kids got older the bullying increased, and for years, I was physically and verbally bullied by other students. Eventually, when I was outed to my parents, I was told I was going to hell. Since I didn't know of any LGBTQIA role models in the media, I fully believed them. Through it all, [in] the arts—acting, singing, dancing—I found my passion and my escape. Not only was it the only place I could truly express myself, but [it was where] I found other kids who were outsiders as well.

My parents were always very supportive about me pursuing artistic endeavors, and I eventually moved to Los Angeles to continue pursuing them professionally. After all the heartache that comes with trying to make it in this industry, including the shut doors in faces, being told I was too femme or too Asian or not white enough, I still struggled to come into my own. It wasn't until the past couple of years when I came to terms with who I really was. After some scary life events, I really dropped my guard finally and embraced myself for who I am.

Life is incredibly short and fragile and I've ultimately concluded that I'd rather spend every day just being my damn self than keep spending all my energy trying to be someone I'm not—and

failing miserably. My hope now is to live my life out and proud to hopefully show some young person who is going through the same things that they are loved. Today, I am continually discovering new things about myself. I have never viewed myself as being strictly within the guidelines of the traditional "male," but I didn't really know how to vocalize it in proper terminology until recently. I have always been nonconforming, a healthy mix of masculine and feminine. In fact, I'm learning that I lean more toward "gender-fluid" since I sort of shift from day to day and I accept ALL pronouns (she/he/they/etc.). I am open to all possibilities, and I am ME. For all others who are discovering themselves, there is a whole world of people that will adore you for being exactly yourself. Queer people can be happy and successful. Don't let anyone tell you any damn different!

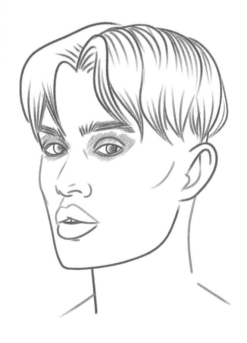

I love all looks. Some days, I'm simple and wear nothing or maybe just a tiny dab of concealer on a blemish. Others, I use a full-coverage foundation, contour and highlight, and sparkle pigment on my eyes. I lean toward a more dewy and natural approach to skin, and I love smoky bold runway-inspired makeup looks that make me feel glamorous. I'm personally not huge on Instagram beauty trends. I like more artistic/timeless looks, but I appreciate it all!

Start with self-care.

First of all, in a world that is actively trying to take rights away from queer people, self-care is an act of political defiance. I start with an almost obsessive skincare routine. I had awful acne growing up and finally got it under control with Accutane. As an adult my skin is very dry, sensitive, and still acne-prone, but controllable. I make sure to use lots of nourishing oils and hydrators that are noncomedogenic and fragrance-free.

New to makeup? No problem.

NYX and Morphe make incredible products that are totally affordable. Morphe eyeshadow palettes go such a long way and won't break your bank. FENTY makes amazing foundations that accurately represent skin tones, and e.l.f. products are actually really great. Don't feel like you have to spend a ton of money to get great results. Also, my favorite Korean foundation is the COSRX blemish spot cover cushion and concealer. It goes on dewy, is super hydrating, and looks natural.

Don't be afraid to experiment!

I personally find myself right in the middle of blurring masculine and feminine vibes, but some days I'm fully a boy with a beard and some days I have a wig on with lashes or any combination thereof.

Don't feel the need to follow the rules of what other people might define as "nonbinary aesthetics." It's all about feeling confident in however you choose to present yourself. If there's one major tip I can give people just starting out with makeup: less is more. Watch lots of YouTube tutorials but take it all with an enormous grain of salt. What you see in those tutorials is meant to look amazing on camera. It's heavy, full-coverage foundations, crazy pigmented multishade shadows, super-dark contour, white highlight, and then overbaked concealers. No one—*no one*—looks good IRL with baked white undereye concealer. It creases and it looks awful.

Start off with minimal product that matches your skin tone (side note: can we all start embracing our actual skin tones please?) and take the time to blend. Pro tip: Don't put liquid products on top of powders. Pro Tip II: If you want a natural look, please wipe the makeup off your hair around your hairline and eyebrows.

Most important, learn to listen to yourself.

Take your time and come out at your own speed. You don't have to share anything you don't want to with the world. Express yourself if it makes *you* feel good. Also, don't be afraid to change your mind! I came out as nonbinary and said I only preferred they/them pronouns, but now I'm finding I like it all! It's okay to change and constantly evolve. You are loved no matter what.

> "I am open to all possibilities, and I am ME."
>
> —CHESTER LOCKHART

LET'S GET IT CLEAR

A history of "cursed skin" and its wild remedies.

In Which the Egyptians Discover Acne

Fun fact: The ancient Egyptians invented acne. Well, the word, at least. According to the Ebers papyrus, an ancient medical scroll dating back to 1500 BCE, the word *aku-t* describes boils, sores, pustules, or any inflamed swelling one might experience. Eventually, aku-t would become the Greek word for "acne," (from the sixth-century term and Greek spelling "acme"), the word we still use today in the Western world.

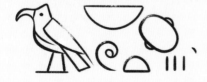

Spoiled Milk and Honey

Speaking of aku-t, the ancient Egyptians were ahead of medical curve when it came to treating pustules. Egyptian physicians used spoiled milk and honey as an effective remedy for pimples. It's even recorded that Cleopatra doused herself with pungent dairy for the sake of clear skin. Sound gross? Sure. But it also worked: milk contains lactic acid, a potent exfoliating ingredient known as an AHA (alpha hydroxy acid), popular in skincare today for sloughing away dead skin cells. As for honey, it's a natural antiseptic with anti-inflammatory properties. Though certainly effective for blackheads and whiteheads, neither work for treating deep, painful cysts, which require benzoyl peroxide or, in extremely severe cases, an Accutane prescription. The teenage king Tutankhamun experienced painful acne during the latter part of his life—archaeologists would discover that he had a face full of cysts along with deep scars.

PUSTULES AND PIMPLES AND PUBERTY, OH MY! TURNS OUT, teens have been picking their pores, leaving behind crater-size scars, and suffering from acne in silence throughout history. Angry, throbbing skin doesn't give AF who you are, where you're from, or what you did (cue Backstreet Boys here), as long as you're an oil-prone human.

Researchers have confirmed that acne in its various forms—the large, itchy or painful red cystic and hormonal acne, and the comedones, papules, and pustules of bacterial acne—and their causes—clogged pores or inflammation, excess oil production, overactive *Cutibacterium acnes* bacteria, genetics—are unique to *Homo sapiens* alone. (Though animals like Fido the French bulldog can produce their own kind of canine-specific acne!) Yet while technology has advanced and information is more accessible as ever, acne remains one of the most misunderstood skin phenomena. Just imagine how confusing it was in ancient times when they didn't have subreddits or forums dedicated to achieving clear skin!

The following is a brief history of desperate quests to ward off acne—some surprisingly effective, others absolutely appalling—and achieve clear, perfect complexions.

750–650 BCE

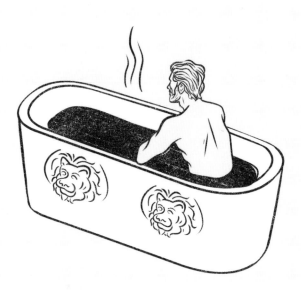

Naked Salt Baths

Of all the subjects he could have recorded, Hesiod, one of the world's first self-proclaimed poets, wrote in-depth about restorative baths. The ancient Greeks thought of warm saunas and hot springs as sacred waters for healing the body. The naturally sulfurous tubs were actually very effective at clearing body acne. Today, dermatologists still prescribe sulfur as a means of drying out excess oil in order to treat acne. And when it comes to salt, experts now say it's great at absorbing impurities and soaking up sebum.

Star Skin

While the Greeks were pretty, er, spot-on when it came to understanding when most would experience acne, the Romans would wish upon a star. Literally. According to physicians under emperor Theodosius the Great, acne could be remedied simply by taking a cloth and wiping pimples away under a shooting star.

Just a Wee Bit More

The Scots in the Highlands thought using urine as an everyday facial cleanser was effective at rinsing away acne, and believed that rubbing a baby's face with a wet diaper could prevent them from developing acne later. The practice was popularized by British naturopath John W. Armstrong, who called it "urine therapy." Some Native American tribes in North America prescribed this as well. While it seems a bit extreme, there's a resurgence of modern-day skincare advocates who swear by this practice, and writers from publications like Refinery29, *Cosmopolitan,* and *Vice* have experimented with using urine to treat acne and dry skin. Their conclusion? It'd probably be safest and most hygienic to stick to our modern treatments.

1 CE ·········· 2 CE ·· 3 CE ·········· 16TH CENTURY ··········

Thy Pole Must Not Be Polished

In 1 AD, Rome's royalty as well as its top gladiators were treated by surgeon-physician, Claudius Galen. The man was considered highly capable at treating most ailments. But his one recommendation for wiping out acne? "Stop masturbating."

Boys 2(CE) Men

Greek writings by physician Aetius Amidenus talk about acne, or "acme," as a "point or spot." Others called acne *tovoot,* which means "the first growth of the beard," referring to puberty and how the blemishes sprout when a boy is transitioning to man. In the seventh century, Paulus Aegineta, another physician, recommended honey for "softer lesions" and soap and honey for pimples that were harder to the touch. Today, synthetic ingredients like benzoyl peroxide and salicylic acid are used for spot treatments.

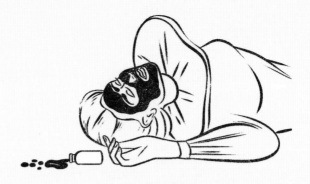

A Treatment to Die For

During the Elizabethan era, an extremely pale, ghostlike complexion indicated wealth and high social status. To get their faces stark white, royals applied thick layers of their favorite cosmetic product, Venetian ceruse (aka Spirits of Saturn), a mixture of lead and vinegar that lasted all day. But it also caused skin conditions like acne. It didn't help that these royals didn't wash their makeup off at night. The court's physicians discovered that mercury (a deadly poison) was effective at both removing Venetian ceruse and treating acne. Mercury was so effective that it burned the blemishes right off *and* killed its users. Today, historians believe ceruse was the culprit behind Queen Elizabeth I's death (see page 70 for more).

1 5 5 8   1 6 0 3   1 6 4 8

I Doo Declare

In Japan's Edo era, geishas and Kabuki actors experienced spots and diseases from using face powders full of zinc and poisonous lead. The latter was dangerous and was said to strip skin off the face. As an alternative, these performers began to turn to a different white substance: bird poop. Called *uguisu no fun,* which literally translates to "nightingale droppings," the natural product effectively painted the skin white, but its enzymes also made it a potent acne-fighting masks. Today, there are still Japanese brands that market bird excrement as a natural alternative to synthetic chemicals.

Abstaining from Acne

A fifteenth-century physician named J. Johnston believed acne was a psychosomatic affliction. That is, he believed the brain was able to create physical ailments. In his opinion, an excessive sex drive was the root cause. In his work *Idea Universae Medicinae Practica,* he described acne as "tiny hard tumours on the skin of the face curdled up of a hard thick juice." He went on to record, "They are about the size of a hemp seed, and they infect young people, who are inclined to venery and fruit-ful, but chast withal and continent." Translated to modern-day English: "Pimples sprout among guys who are horny and alone."

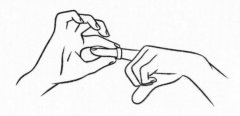

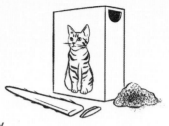

Tie the Knot

Theories of excessive sexual activity, thoughts, or self-love as the cause of acne continued into the seventeenth and eighteenth centuries. Some physicians went so far as to prescribe marriage as a cure. But what about those who were married and still experienced acne? Well, those were the ones who had an "abnormal sex life."

Pretty Kitty

Back before YouTuber and beauty mogul Michelle Phan became a household name, she was the original beauty vlogger providing tips to the masses. In 2013, she had a viral video that made international headlines after she used kitty litter as a face mask. Yep, Phan claimed the mixture of litter and aloe vera made her skin soft, pores shrunken, and acne obsolete. That's because the litter has bits of clay in it, which she claimed made it an effective—and frugal—$2 face mask.

1800–1900 ·········· 2013 ······· PRESENT DAY!

Today, acne treatments are as obsessed-over as ever. There are pimple patches that range from those with hyaluronic acids that soothe the pores and soak up pus to those with dissolving microneedles used to prick and treat cysts. For those who want medication, there are several direct-to-consumer businesses that prescribe acne-fighting antibiotics over the web. The fastest treatment is a visit to the dermatologist for a cortisone shot, one that will dissolve even the angriest of pimples in mere minutes. But perhaps the most inspiring treatment of all is no treatment at all. In our modern age, there's been an acne-acceptance movement, one that promotes celebrating your skin, pimples and all. Who says acne can't be beautiful, too?

Everything you've ever wanted to ask about acne.

If skincare's a journey, acne is an entire three-part saga full of ups and downs, with unexpected twists and turns. That's because when it comes to these curious pustules and cysts, there's no one reason that they come to destroy your pores. You may have just read all of the *creative* ways people throughout history have endeavored to banish their angry spots, but it's time to talk to a modern-day expert: Dr. Y. Claire Chang, a board-certified cosmetic dermatologist in New York City.

So how is acne formed?!

Many reasons—from your pores getting clogged with dead skin cells, oil, makeup to other impurities—it gets complicated. Bacteria, most notably *Cutibacterium acnes,* builds up within these pores to activate skin inflammation. The pore can then rupture, releasing its contents and bacteria, which triggers your body to attack it. This results in an inflammatory response leading to the formation of inflammatory acne lesions, like papules, pustules, and cysts.

So there are different forms of acne?

Acne can be broadly categorized into two camps: non-inflammatory and inflammatory lesions.

Non-inflammatory lesions include comedones, more commonly known as whiteheads and blackheads. Comedones occur when pores or hair follicles become clogged with oil, dead skin cells, and other impurities. Closed comedones, or whiteheads, are flesh-colored or whitish 1- to 3-millimeter papules. Open comedones, aka blackheads, are similar in appearance but have a dark center due to an opening at their surface. Inflammatory lesions are those that are red and inflamed.

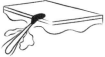

BLACKHEAD   WHITEHEAD

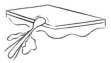

Inflammatory lesions include papules (small tender red bumps), pustules (white or yellow pus-filled bumps), cysts (larger firm red bumps), and nodules (painful, deeper lumps). Papules and pustules are raised red lesions that are 2 to 5 millimeters in diameter. Pustules are filled with white or yellow material (pus) due to inflammation. These are tempting to touch, but should not be popped or squeezed.

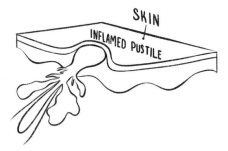

Each person can have several types of acne at the same time. Acne scarring occurs in up to 90 percent of acne patients ("Acne and resulting acne scarring can cause significant distress, anxiety, and reduced self-esteem in patients.") and is characterized by blemishes, atrophic scarring, and hypertrophic (raised above the skin) scarring.

The causes?

Ugh, there are many. These include hormones, stress, diet, and medications. "The cause of acne is complex, including abnormal buildup of skin cells, oil production, blocked pores, bacterial growth, and inflammation," Dr. Chang says.

So how do you get rid of it?

First off: prevention.

"Especially if acne is a recurrent problem, you should be on a maintenance regimen to prevent new acne lesions from occurring in the first place," says Dr. Chang. "I recommend consulting your local dermatologist to figure out the best acne regimen for you. Everyone responds differently to individual acne treatments, and it takes commitment and patience to determining the best regimen."

But there are many over-the-counter remedies you can try!

The following are wonder ingredients, according to Dr. Chang:

Salicylic acid is available in drugstores as a cleanser, toner, lotion, and spot treatment. Salicylic acid is a beta hydroxy acid that works as a keratolytic. It is more oil-soluble than an AHA, allowing it to penetrate deeper into the skin and the pores to remove dead skin cells. Salicylic acid helps exfoliate the skin and keep the pores clear. It works best for mild acne and comedonal acne (whiteheads and blackheads).

Benzoyl peroxide has anti-inflammatory and antibacterial properties that can help treat inflammation and kill acne-causing bacteria. Benzoyl peroxide can help prevent and treat inflammatory acne, including those pesky red bumps and cysts. Benzoyl peroxide can be used effectively alongside other topicals, including topical antibiotics.

Azelaic acid is a dicarboxylic acid that can be found over the counter. Azelaic acid can help fight acne-causing bacteria and inflammation. It also gently increases skin cell turnover. Azelaic acid also helps with rosacea and hyperpigmentation, making it ideal for those who have acne rosacea and acne scars.

WHEN THE GOING GETS TOUGH, STICK WITH IT!

"A common mistake is trying new skincare products for one week and then giving up, or jumping from one regimen to another," Dr. Chang says. "Patience is key—it can take six to eight weeks of continued use for topical acne treatments to start working."

IF WORSE COMES TO WORST, ASK FOR PRESCRIPTION MEDICATION.

Treatments can be divided into topical and oral therapies. The type of treatment needed depends on the patient, the type of acne lesions they have, and the severity of their acne. There are also over-the-counter retinoids like Differin, which no longer need prescriptions.

Topical treatments can come in the form of cleansers, toners, creams, masks, and spot treatments. One of the gold standards of acne therapy is topical retinoid treatment. Retinoids are vitamin A derivatives that have been shown to normalize skin cell turnover and fight inflammation. Retinoids are effective in treating both noninflammatory and inflammatory acne lesions. As for oral medications, many dermatologists prescribe isotrentinoin, an oral medicine, which seems to have effective results, although results have shown it can cause depression or be toxic for pregnant women. To get a prescription, one must get their blood taken every month, and have monthly check-ins with their dermatologists. Of course, consult your dermatologist, read further studies, and side effects to see if this is best for you.

AT-HOME TIPS . . . AND MORE!
- Ice your acne to help calm inflammation.
- Use a red LED light to kill bacteria.
- Stick on acne patches to slurp up excess fluid and sebum.
- Keep an eye on your lifestyle, and make sure you're eating a good diet, getting enough sleep, and managing your stress levels.
- Wash your face regularly and use noncomedogenic makeup.

BUT MOST IMPORTANT . . .

"Remember never to touch or irritate your pimples," Dr. Chang says. "Popping, picking, or squeezing your pimple can trigger more trauma and inflammation, eventually leading to more scarring."

MAX FACTOR

(1 8 7 7 - 1 9 3 8)

*The godfather of modern cosmetics used
makeup as survival.*

WE'RE IN AN ERA OF BEAUTY BRAND ABUNDANCE, WHICH SOME would argue is borderline excessive. From thousands of custom foundations, concealers, BB creams, and color cosmetics like lip glosses, eyeshadows, mascaras, and more, the biggest conundrum consumers face today is being bombarded with too much choice.

So it's difficult to imagine a time when cosmetics weren't available commercially at all. But a century ago, the only makeup available were clumsy concoctions made exclusively for the wealthy. And even those weren't very good, with their difficult applications, toxic ingredients, and unrealistic shades.

Of course, all that changed when Max Factor came along. He'd democratize cosmetics by providing affordable products to the masses—and even coin the term "makeup" itself. He was so successful that his eponymous brand is still thriving today.

While this godfather of beauty was known as a makeup artist to the stars, his story is hardly one of overnight success.

....

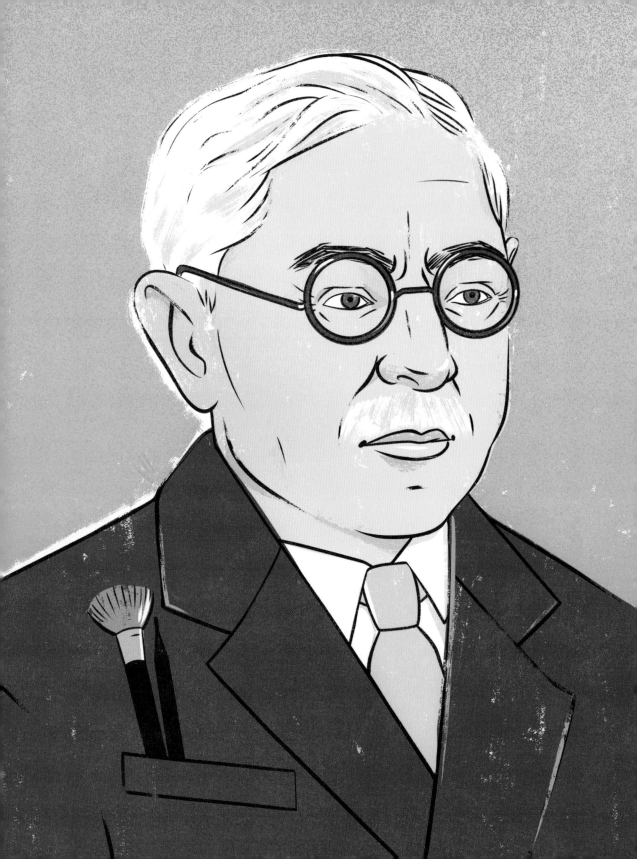

Maksymilian Faktorowicz had no other choice but to pretend he was dying. After serving four years in the Russian Army, he had found himself working for the Russian royal family as their go-to hair-and-makeup artist. "All my attention went to their individual needs by showing them how to enhance their good points and conceal the less good," he later recalled. To say the Russian royals were needy is an understatement. The hours were so long and the women so fussy, the beautician was allotted a mere one hour to himself a week. Which he certainly took advantage of—he was not only able to find someone to marry, he ended up having three children, all without the royals knowing. But as a Polish immigrant *and* a Jew during a time in which violent anti-Semitism was rising around the country, his only chance at survival was to flee Russia.

One day, after hearing of Maksymilian's secret family, an ally within the Russian military offered his support in fleeing the country. But the stylist would first need the royal family's consent to cross the border, which seemed impossible, given how much they depended on him.

So the beautician did what he knew best: he used makeup. But instead of slathering himself in beautiful rouges or creams, he put on yellows and grays to make himself look sickly and sallow. He did an exceptional job, because the moment the family saw his poor complexion, they suggested he leave immediately for Carlsbad, a city in Bohemia in what is now the Czech Republic, where the sick would go to recover.

When he arrived in Carlsbad, he met up with his family, and the four rushed toward a seaport hundreds of miles away. There, the family boarded the S.S. *Moltka,* a ship headed to America, the land of the free.

At Ellis Island, Maksymilian Faktorowicz became "Max Factor." He didn't mind the liberty taken by the American border official, though, thinking of the change as a means of sloughing his old identity and transforming it into an American form. He settled his family in St. Louis, Missouri, where his father and brother had emigrated. To survive in those early days, he sold homemade rouges and creams at the 1904 World's Fair. It wasn't an easy way to make a living, but it was still a start.

After his first wife died in 1906 and he discovered that his business partner had stolen his life savings, he decided to start a new life and headed for California. He set up his own business in Los Angeles, selling wigs and stage makeup. A sign hung outside the store read: "Max Factor's Antiseptic Hair Store. Toupees made to order. High grade work." He became transfixed by the actors who would walk by his shop every evening. Each looked absolutely ghoulish—but not in a good way—their faces were grayish, lathered in grease, Vaseline, lard, flour, and cold cream. Some took it even further, ruddying their complexions with paprika and brick dust, concoctions that were supposed to mimic a natural, flesh-colored look.

Soon he became a distributor of greasepaint, a greasy, waxy, thick, oil-based makeup these actors used for their jobs. Not only was the formula unstable (with time, the product would change the color of the wearer's skin), it was difficult to make it look like real skin onscreen. And it was impossible to work with: it creased whenever actors would emote, and would glide off their faces, melting under the harsh lights on set.

Max could do better. In 1914, he concocted his own version, which he called "flexible greasepaint." It was blendable and layerable, and looked more natural. It was so effective that he was tasked by Hollywood studios with creating twelve different shade ranges. He tested the colors on his first clients, silent-film actor Charlie Chaplin and cowboy star Tom Mix. While the two initially thought makeup was "too sissy," they would not only return, but ensure Max became their personal makeup artist.

His name began to circulate around Hollywood. He was nimble, a master problem-solver, and was known for creating ingenious, out-of-the-box solutions for his many clients. When the actress Phyllis Haver wanted sexier roles, he sewed her false eyelashes from human hair. When the actor Rudolph Valentino wanted to step outside his villain typecasting, Max created yellow makeup to lighten his skin. When Joan Crawford needed an extreme makeover, he overdrew her lips using a technique he would call "the smear," adding more depth and beauty to her rather plain face. The look would become her signature.

As Hollywood evolved, so did Max's makeup. With better black-and-white film being introduced, he created entirely new formulations to reflect indoor set lights. Called "panchromatic makeup," it was "horrifying to look at in daylight," but worked well in a controlled environment, absorbing the light emitted from high-wattage bulbs. As Technicolor films became more commonplace, Max's makeup continued to become more subtle. His foundations were so good, actresses were rumored to steal them from film sets.

With this in mind, he decided he'd put his entrepreneurial skills to work. If actresses were clamoring for his makeup, why wouldn't the general public? And so, he took cosmetics "out of the stars' dressing rooms and into the drugstore." It was around this time that he coined the term "makeup"—short for "to make-up one's face"—and debuted a hit product called Society Make-Up, a foundation that would hold from day to night. He'd go on to create iterations of this—his most successful coverage makeup ever was Pan-Cake, available in twelve shades. It was foundation in a compact, caked form that came with a circular tin encasement. One only needed to dip a wet sponge to activate the product, which was rich and thick, with a matte finish. It sold out everywhere.

"YOU ARE NOT BORN GLAMOROUS. GLAMOUR IS CREATED."

—MAX FACTOR

Of course, Max never stopped. He'd go on to invent other commercial products that became necessities for the actors he worked with, as well as for laypeople. Soon, other easy-to-apply cosmetics inventions debuted in drugstores, including eyeshadows, eyebrow pencils, mascara, lipstick, lip gloss, and more. As Max became a commercial success, he'd be honored for his many important contributions to the film industry. In 1929, he was awarded an honorary Oscar, and even received a star on the Hollywood Walk of Fame.

By the end of his life in 1938, Max Factor had built an incredible beauty empire. In under two decades, the business launched globally, eventually becoming a multimillion-dollar business. Today, the brand is owned by the beauty conglomerate Coty Inc., and remains as popular as ever.

Max shaped the modern beauty industry we know today, but his understanding of beauty was also a key to open the door of acceptance during a time of rising anti-Semitism. "You are not born glamorous," he would later say. "Glamour is created." For Max, the same sentiment rang true for success, and for survival.

BLACK BEAUTY BRANDS BROKE BARRIERS

A History

RIHANNA'S 2017 LAUNCH OF FENTY BEAUTY COULD HAVE BEEN just like any other celebrity cosmetics brand—for years, stars have been shelling out their names along with products to make a quick buck. But this was Rihanna—she's an icon. And FENTY Beauty isn't just a beauty brand—it's part of a cultural movement.

Rihanna follows a long legacy of Black beauty moguls who've built multimillion-dollar cosmetics companies over the past century, including Madam C. J. Walker, America's first self-made female millionaire. (She's the subject of the Netflix miniseries *Self Made,* where actress Octavia Spencer plays the late beauty mogul.) "Madam Walker's Wonderful Hair Grower" beat all odds to find resounding commercial success. But Madam C. J. Walker and Rihanna weren't alone. Black beauty-brand owners have been pushing white-centric boundaries since decades before Rihanna's Gloss Bomb even hit shelves . . .

An Overton Night Sensation

The first cosmetics brand for Black Americans was started by a Black man. Born enslaved, Anthony Overton was an ambitious young person who set his sights on higher education. He graduated from law school and later became a judge.

But after years serving on courts, he realized there was a significant blank space in the market: cosmetics for Black women. And so with $2,000 (roughly $50,000 today) in his savings account, he quit his day job and founded the Overton Hygienic Company. He'd go on to patent his cosmetics formulas, creating a line of makeup ranging from powders to extracts. So popular were his products, he received orders from around the world, including, Liberia, Egypt, and Japan. By 1927, his company employed over four hundred door-to-door salesmen, with an annual profit of $1 million.

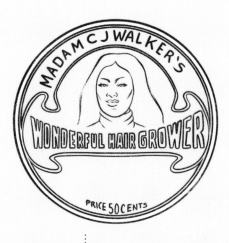

1867–1919   1869–1957   1898–1946

Self Made

Madam C. J. Walker was the first female self-made American millionaire (as seen in the Netflix series). A daughter of slaves, Walker was the first in her family to be born free. She found work in St. Louis as a laundress, but knew she was meant for more.

She enrolled in Annie Turnbo Malone's Poro College and was eventually hired as an employee of Poro Products. While a salesman for the brand, she decided she'd develop her own product line. According to a biography, the ingredients came to her in a dream. They included petrolatum, coconut oil, beeswax, sulfur, and perfume, among others. Called the Wonderful Hair Grower, it was marketed as preventing stress to the scalp. Soon, her hair grower would surpass even that of her former employer, and her empire would cement itself in American history.

Keep It Growing

Annie Turnbo Malone had a knack for hair—she styled her sisters' and would give beauty tips to strangers. Her eye for style led her to develop a hair care line for Black women. She understood that to be accepted as a Black woman by the white communities and industries in the 1800s, one had to put an extra emphasis on their appearance.

Malone faced racism and sexism, but would still create a beauty empire. She began concocting ingredients in her own home, and eventually bottled them up to sell en masse. Her best-selling product at the time was Hair Grower, a formula that was marketed to improve scalp health and promote hair growth. With the proceeds, she was able to start a cosmetics school called Poro College, which transitioned into a line of Poro products, including lipsticks, face powders, cold creams.

The Young and Beautiful

At a time when depictions of Black Americans were stereotypical and blatantly racist, Valmor Products Co., founded by Hungarian American Morton Neumann, capitalized on the lack of self-care and beauty products for Black consumers. The entrepreneur focused on producing Black hair creams and face powders, in addition to perfumes. Valmor's products were themed around romance, with products like Kiss Me Again mouthwash and Hold Your Man perfume. Customers also purchased the brand's skin-lightening and hair-straightening products—this, decades before the Black Is Beautiful campaign. (For more on the "Black Is Beautiful" campaign, see below.) But what made this brand historic was how it employed mostly Black Americans, from its sales team to its graphic design team. It was illustrator Charles C. Dawson, an advocate for equality, who'd sketch Black Americans on its packaging who were far from racist stereotypes: they were glamorous, beautiful, youthful, and chic.

1920 · 1926 · 1950s–1970s

History Rih-peats

Though Rihanna is incomparable, there are historians that tout 1920s star Anita Patti Brown as someone who had a similar career path. Brown was a popular soprano opera singer known as "the Bronze Tetrazzini" and a "globe-trotting prima donna." The artist toured across the United States, South America, and the West Indies before deciding to create her own beauty brand, Patti's Beauty Emporium, which she used her celebrity to advertise. The mail-order business shipped out everything from skincare products to fragrances, and even her own signature "La Traviata" face powder.

Black Is Beautiful

Since colonial times, American beauty standards have been based on a Eurocentric lens. From that stemmed racist notions that Black people and their natural features—skin color, facial features, hair—were inherently ugly. The Black Is Beautiful movement encouraged Black people everywhere to embrace their African features, to stop straightening hair or lightening their skin.

Hoyt W. Fuller observed in 1968: "Across the country, young black men and women have been infected with a fever of affirmation. They are saying, 'We are black and beautiful.'" The "think black, buy black" slogan also arose during this time, catapulting to popularity during a protest against the opening of a white-owned wig shop in New York City's Harlem.

"Fair" Trade

Johnson Publishing Company, established in Chicago by John and Eunice Johnson, created the Ebony Fashion Fair. It was a traveling roadshow of sorts, mixing entertainment, fashion, and onstage performances, in addition to selling goods for their Black American audiences. The show hit thirty cities and operated for fifty-one years. On one stop at a show, Eunice Johnson noticed how the Black models on the runway would have to mix their foundations because they had trouble finding products that matched their skin tones. Out of necessity, Johnson created Fashion Fair Cosmetics to address the needs of Black consumers by providing concentrated pigments in deeper skin tones. Fashion Fair would become the first big brand that was Black-owned, established before conglomerates like Estée Lauder. The brand was touted by *Fortune* magazine as being the biggest Black-owned beauty brand in the world.

1960s · · · 1973 · · · 1994

A Different Shade

The civil rights movement created more equal opportunities for people. In terms of the beauty industry, it desegregated makeup counters. In 1961, this forced major beauty brands from Avon to Maybelline to start catering to Black customers. Half a dozen makeup brands for more diverse skin tones debuted, and Avon used Black models in ads it placed in *Ebony* magazine. One of these models was Tracey "Africa" Norman, the first Black trans woman model, who'd go on to land an exclusive contract with Clairol as well.

Business Model

Before it was normal for models to become their own brands, there was Iman. She launched IMAN, her makeup brand, to meet the needs of people from all backgrounds. "As a model, I had to play chemist and mix and match foundations to find a skin tone suitable for me," she once said to *Time* magazine. "A well-known brand may have six foundations total, whereas I have over 30 foundations just for women of color." Soon the brand launched at places like Target, Duane Reade, Walgreens, and Walmart, among others, to better represent their Black and Brown customers. By 2010, the company was generating $25 million annually.

Flea Market Success

Lisa Price started selling her beauty products in her Brooklyn neighborhoods' flea markets and fairs. Her creams and ointments were ultra-soothing and became a hit from word-of-mouth marketing. It wasn't until she opened Carol's Daughter as a boutique, and later opened up its e-commerce in 2000, that the business really took off. Thanks to a boost in sales from the brand appearing on *The Oprah Winfrey Show,* Carol's Daughter became a multimillion-dollar business. Soon, Lisa was getting attention from investors like Will Smith and Jada Pinkett Smith and Jay-Z. The brand was then sold to L'Oréal in October of 2014. Others, like Shea Moisture and Juvia's Place, to name just a few, would follow suit.

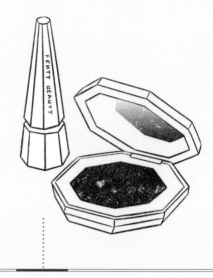

2000 .... **2017**

FENTY Beauty

Rihanna, in partnership with LVHM, debuted a revolutionary brand that put diversity and inclusivity at its forefront, in its campaigns *and* in its products. Its foundation came in forty unique shades, which sold out at Sephora on their first day—the deepest skin tone shades went first. After the launch of forty foundation shades, FENTY Beauty outdid itself and added another ten shades to its Pro Filt'r line.

The legacy of FENTY's overnight success will be lasting. (Months later, Kylie Cosmetics, founded by Kylie Jenner, announced that it would expand its own foundation range to thirty shades, and other brands have followed suit.) While there have been Black beauty pioneers before the entertainer and entrepreneur, never has such an inclusive brand reached a global audience, proving that inclusivity pays dividends, and that a beauty brand can truly push culture in the right direction.

Today, many more Black-owned beauty brands have thrived, including men's grooming brand Bevel, women's shaving brand OUI the People, the cosmetics brands UOMA Beauty and Coloured Raine, and many more. In 2020, Sharon Chuter, founder of UOMA, challenged beauty brands to reveal how many Black employees worked in their businesses. Called #pulluporshutup, the social media campaign pushed brands to become more accountable and hire people from diverse backgrounds.

REMOVE YOUR MAKEUP THE RIGHT WAY

Take it all off like a pro.

Putting on makeup can take up a good chunk of your day, depending on your look. But just because you've put so much energy into painting your face doesn't mean you shouldn't be putting in the same amount of energy removing it. Nothing's worse than going to bed with a full face of foundation, eyes globbed with mascara, or lips still lined. Not only will it get your sheets dirty, it'll most likely clog your pores, which can lead to breakouts, acne, or bacterial infections—yikes! Here are the best (and easiest) ways to remove your makeup in just minutes.

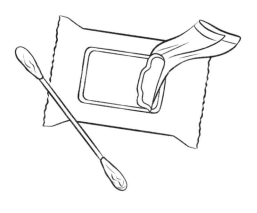

1. START WITH AN OIL CLEANSER OR A MAKEUP WIPE.

Oil is the only ingredient that can trap oil. So to really get into your pores to remove makeup, you'll want a good oil cleanser, makeup wipe with oil, or balm. If you're using a cleanser, simply place a quarter-size amount in your palms, then massage it onto your face. After around 15 to 30 seconds, wash it away with water. If you're using a wipe, use both sides to get as much product off as possible. Most of your makeup should be removed at this point.

2. DOUBLE CLEANSE NEXT.

An oil cleanser will wash off most of your makeup—but not all of it. For your next step, use your favorite foam or gel cleanser. Don't forget your eyes, either, gently cleansing them. If it burns, rinse your eyes immediately with water.

3. MICELLAR WATER IS YOUR NEW BFF.

If you still have makeup on at this point, it's probably your eye makeup, with your eyeliner and mascara holding on for dear life. If this is the case, take a cotton pad, drench it with micellar water, and gently wipe your eyes. If that still isn't working, take a Q-tip, soak it in micellar water, and swipe it across your eye's waterline. Do so until all the product is removed.

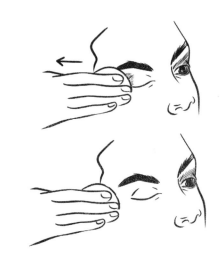

4. SKINCARE ISN'T TO BE SKIPPED!

After you finish removing all makeup with these steps, you'll want to proceed with your skincare. If you're *not* down for a 10-step K-beauty regimen (no judgment!), try a toner, which will balance out your skin's pH and soften your skin, followed with a cream. Two products, and you're done for the night!

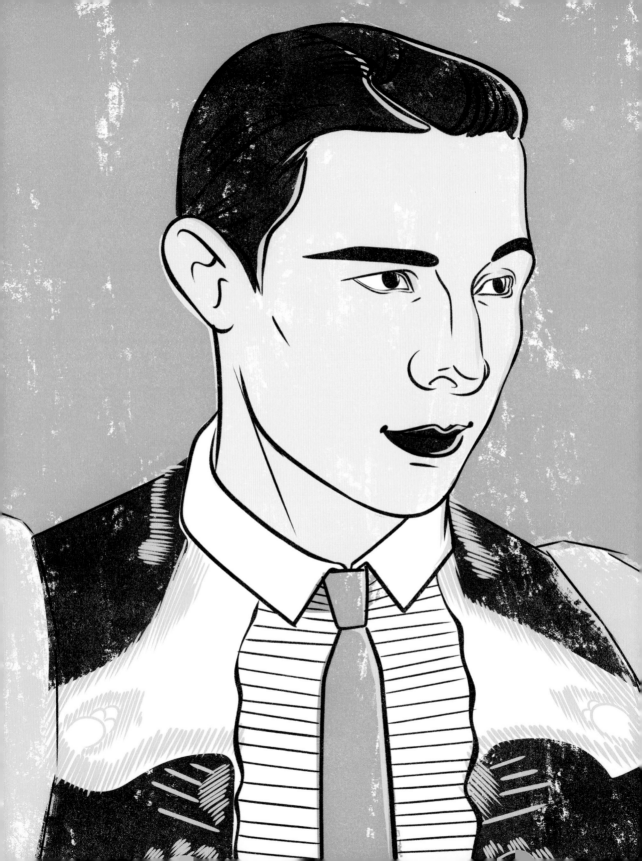

RUDOLPH VALENTINO

(1895-1926)

The pretty boy who knocked out his rivals.

TODAY, OUR HONOR IS WON OR LOST ON THE TWITTER BAT-tlefield. But a century before our thumbs became our biggest defenders, beefs were handled inside a boxing ring. Dishonor your friend? Here's an uppercut. Offend your rival? Let's take this outside. Say something stupid? That deserves a swing to the head.

And a fight there would be, after a *Chicago Tribune* reporter walked into a men's bathroom to discover a pink face-powder dispenser, and blamed it on the influence of Rudolph Valentino, aka the "Latin Lover."

"Homo Americanus! Why didn't someone quietly drown Rudolph Guglielmo, alias Valentino, years ago?" wrote the journalist. "Hollywood is a national school of masculinity. Rudy, the beautiful gardener's boy, is the prototype of the American male. Hell's bells. Oh, sugar."

He wasn't the only one who took offense at the Italian star and his aesthetics. As America's first major celebrity crush, one who would "single-handedly change the way generations of men and women thought about sex and seduction," Valentino had a way with both women and men. He seduced the former and challenged the latter. One of the most visible men in Hollywood during this era, he became famous through his roles in 1921's *The Four Horsemen of the Apocalypse,* one of the first films to rake in over $1 million at the box office, and 1926's *The Sheik,* in which he starred as the lead heartthrob. His darker Italian features were considered exotic and his mannerisms altogether romantic. But it was his makeup, which smoothed out his pores and made his nose seem extra thin and his lips more luscious, that caused an uproar in greater male society.

The cisgender white men of America felt threatened that they were being eclipsed by a foreign entity. So for years, the media chipped away at Valentino, questioning the actor's sexuality, emasculating him, in the hopes that he'd one day just up and disappear. They went after his aesthetics—his painted face, the earrings he wore in films, his long lashes, his "patent leather hair," giving him the nickname The Latin Lover. In turn, men who mimicked his strapping and trendsetting style were called "Vaselinos." But Valentino's slicked-back style still caught on, and reportedly inspired hordes of men to run out and buy shiny brilliantine, a scented oil that made hair look glossy.

By today's standard, these editorials would be nothing more than a troll's comments on some celebrity's Instagram page. But at the time, the offensive columns made national headlines. The *Chicago Tribune* op-ed was particularly grievous, as it came at a time when Valentino had just become a household name. Having no other choice but to defend his honor and career, Valentino did what old-school men did best: challenged the writer to an open duel.

In an interview with the *New York Times,* Valentino said he wanted to prove "in typically American fashion, for I am an American citizen, which is the better man." It wasn't a publicity stunt, he clarified; rather, it would end public discussion of his masculinity once and for all.

In an open letter, he called the author of the op-ed a "coward," and said he wanted "an opportunity to demonstrate to you that the wrist under a slave bracelet may snap a real fist into your sagging jaw." The reporter never answered Valentino's invitation and blamed illness for his inability to take up the challenge. While he was waiting for a response, Valentino took the ensuing publicity in stride, getting photographed shirtless, his biceps bulging and his chest chiseled. He was serious about this match, and took boxing lessons from the heavyweight champion Jack Dempsey, training in front of cameras. Talk about milking his moment in the spotlight!

PRETTY BOYS CAN and DO CLAP BACK.

Months later, still having no luck with getting the reporter to agree to a fight, Jack asked his friend Frank O'Neil, a sportswriter, for help. He decided to volunteer to take on Valentino in the ring. "Cut the crap. I don't buy it, and neither does anyone else," he said, doubting Valentino's physicality.

The two eventually met on a Chicago rooftop, with reporters and photographers capturing every move. When the boxing match began, O'Neil clocked Valentino on his left chin. The Italian actor then punched his opponent with a mean left jab. O'Neil dropped to the floor. Apologizing for what he'd done, Valentino helped O'Neil to his feet. "That boy has a punch like a mule's kick," the reporter later said in defeat. "I'd sure hate to have him sore at me."

Months later, whisperings about the star's sexuality and masculinity finally began to fade. In retrospect, we now see that the Italian actor was doing more than just flexing his machismo and physical strength—he was trying to "teach [him] to respect a man even though he happens to prefer to keep his face clean." In other words, masculinity does not exclude beauty, and this pretty boy would not tolerate homophobia, xenophobia, and racism. Yes, pretty boys can and do clap back.

If you have hair, chances are you've tried parting it at one point in your life. But according to Hollywood's most sought-out groomer, Kristan Serafino, you may have been doing it wrong. Serafino is the genius behind the godly coifs of the industry's hottest stars, including Ryan Reynolds, Jake Gyllenhaal, and Robert Pattinson. The one factor that makes or breaks a good hairstyle? Getting that part just right. And on the side is where it's at: "Parting your hair to the left or right makes a huge difference to your face," says Serafino. "It may not seem like it's a big deal, but parting it the wrong way can be a change for the worse."

Here's Serafino's play-by-play for finding and styling your side part. As a bonus, she shares how she keeps her A-list clients looking their best all day long.

FIND YOUR PART

The easiest trick in detecting your hair's natural part is the forward-and-back method. Serafino says to comb your fingers backward in your hair and then move it from left to right. "Your hair will fall in the direction that it grows in. When that happens, you know that that's the way you should go." If you're still having trouble, try locating your cowlick. Pretty much everyone has one. The cowlick is the outward spiral of hair located near the back of your head (where your bald spot is). When you look at it in a mirror, you can find which way it naturally grows. If the spiral grows clockwise, comb to the left. If it grows counterclockwise, comb to the right. If you have two cowlicks, that means you have the freedom to comb whichever way you want, you handsome man, you!

WHEN IN DOUBT, ASK YOUR BARBER

If you're still confused, ask your local barber—they won't mind. "You wouldn't believe how many guys are amazed when I tell them their true higher part calling," says Serafino. "Their lives are changed."

A LITTLE GOES A LONG WAY

Whether it's clay, pomade, gel, or a hybrid of them all, chances are you're using way too much product. Which is understandable, especially if you have unruly hair that doesn't seem to stay in place. But still, "Less is more," Serafino says. "You only need a pea-sized to a dime-sized amount." Product can weigh down your hair so let your hair's natural fibers and oils do work, too. And yes, a small amount even works well for curly or wavy hair (like for her client, *Riverdale* actor Charles Melton, whose waves are wow-inducing).

DON'T PALM IT

It's natural to want to take product and rub it in between your palms before placing it in your hair. The thought process is that it'll warm up and activate the product. Instead, the product soaks into your palms and doesn't necessarily transfer into your hair. "I can't tell you the number of guys who do this and find that no product is actually going in," Serafino says. "There's no product going to your head." Instead, rub product between your fingers and massage it in from the root upward. This is a tip she gives clients like Robert Pattinson and Daniel Craig. Let your fingers act as combs, going from root to tip, and allow the product to do its job.

START IN THE BACK

Instinctively, guys want to put product in their hair from front to back. But that's not the most effective strategy. Instead, put product in from back to front. "Most of your hair is in the back of your head, so putting products front to back means you're weighing it down," Serafino shares. Put that together with sweat, natural oils, and the elements, and you'll end up with floppy, droopy hair. "For thinning hair, this accentuates how thin it is," she says. Another reason to start back to front is to distribute the product evenly over your head. Starting from the back and working toward the front will coat your hair fibers evenly.

GO AGAINST THE GRAIN

For the best volume? Style your hair against the way it's naturally growing out. If it grows to the left, lift the hair, add product, and style it to the right. "Lift the hair with your pinky, separate the sections, spray it with a product, and style in the opposite direction," Serafino says. Use a blow-dryer if you want to achieve more drama. The result: the volume of your dreams, and the perfect part.

COMB YOUR FINGERS BACKWARD IN YOUR HAIR AND THEN MOVE IT FROM LEFT TO RIGHT. YOUR HAIR WILL FALL IN THE DIRECTION THAT IT GROWS IN.

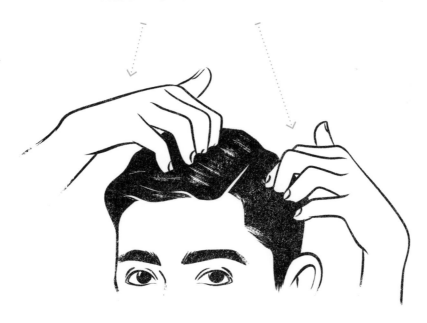

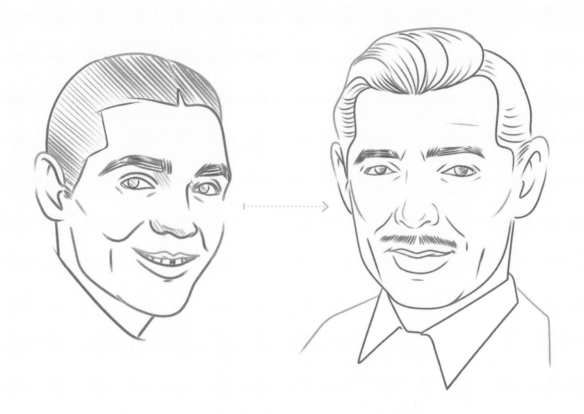

CLARK GABLE

(1901-1960)

Mask of masculinity.

THERE'S NO STAR WHO BETTER PERSONIFIES OLD HOLLYWOOD style, elegance, and sex appeal than Clark Gable. Remembered for his debonair flair, signature pencil mustache, slick side-parted hair, and his roles in movies like the infamously racist *Gone With the Wind,* the actor is still revered as the quintessential American vision of masculinity.

But when he was growing up in the small country town of Cadiz, Ohio, Clark was unremarkable. Tall and gangly, with a gap-toothed smile and floppy ears, he blended in with the other farm boys in town. But his big ambitions stood out. Obsessed with performance and thinking he was much more than what his small town could offer, he soon left his childhood behind to pursue his big dreams in Hollywood.

He made it to Portland, Oregon, where he sold neckties by day and was a theater geek by night. There he met an acting coach by the name of Josephine Dillon, who'd eventually become his first wife. Eighteen years his senior, she was more of a guide than a lover, providing him with free tips on how to become more of a viable leading man. Slouch less, speak more confidently, she instructed. Be more Hollywood.

When they made the move to Hollywood, Clark would discover that he still didn't stand out. Far from landing any leading roles, he was cast as an extra in films like 1925's *The Merry Widow* and *The Plastic Age.* He made his way with a few speaking parts as minor characters in a few other movies before deciding to pack his bags and try his luck in New York City, where he hoped the Great White Way might lead him to Broadway stardom. In the Big Apple is where he found roles onstage—*and* a new wife. He eventually divorced Josephine and married a Texas socialite named—wait for it—Maria Franklin Prentiss Lucas Langham. Like Josephine, she was much older than him—twenty years, to be exact—but she was loaded.

Clark ultimately left a mediocre career on Broadway in the early 1930s and made his way back to California . . . where he was told he was still "too elephant-eared and unattractive" to be a leading man (this coming from MGM's own studio bigwig).

At the time, the All-American aesthetic was blond hair and blue eyes, so the darker-haired Clark took the roles of villains in flicks like *Night Nurse* for years. He was a little more tan than other actors of the era, and a little rougher around the edges, and audiences began to be drawn not to only his booming voice and his natural charisma, but to how different he looked from every other cookie-cutter, fair-skinned Aryan man. Even MGM changed their minds about the actor. Seeing that he was becoming bankable, they decided they wanted to invest in his future.

At the time, actors were contracted to individual movie studios, which meant the studios had their own roster of talent for their own projects. And MGM was desperate for its own leading man. But to ensure a return on their investment, they needed Clark to get an even more extreme Hollywood makeover. That started with sending him to a dentist to fix his gum disease, pull out his rotting teeth, and fit him with pearly white dentures. Then they forced him to the gym to add some bulk. The salons beautified his grayish complexion so it became more sanguine. Groomers plucked and tweezed every stray hair from his eyebrows and finessed his facial hair. They instructed him to grow out his hair and comb it to the side with shiny pomade, in what would become his signature look.

Yet aesthetics weren't everything. The studio also needed him to *live* the lifestyle of a leading man, the American ideal of ultimate masculinity. More hypermasculine, tough-and-gruff man, less sensitive Midwesterner. So they bought him a new wardrobe, brought in a tutor to teach him how to fish and "be an outdoorsman," and pushed him to live a more lavish lifestyle. At the time, America was obsessed with the outdoors, the ultimate symbol of man being closer to his innate self, exploring the wild. In only a few months, Clark was almost unrecognizable, his old skin replaced with something new.

And all of this worked. His new macho attitude and tough demeanor made him into a sensation with all genders. Soon men were emulating Clark's slicked-back side part and growing their own pencil mustaches, puffing out their chests and adopting his hypermasculine demeanor. Clark would go on to be a legend in American cinema. He'd eventually be awarded "Best Actor" at the Oscars for *It Happened One Night,* and continued his leading man status with movies like *San Francisco, Test Pilot,* and *Boom Town.* He inspired countless actors and everyday folks—even today, you can find hundreds of articles and thousands of how-to guides on how to achieve his style, how to emulate his version of manhood. Ironically, they're following the lead of a man whose image of masculinity was entirely constructed by a man who was more than willing to alter his image, erase his roots, and give into Hollywood for the sake of fame and fortune. Damn, was he good at acting.

SHI PEI PU

(1938-2009)

The spy who loved me.

LIKE MANY ROMANCES, THIS ONE WAS TOXIC.

Beijing, 1964: It's been over ten years since the Korean War, and China is undergoing its Cultural Revolution. Winter in Beijing is frigid, inspiring singles to seek out lovers even if just to help keep them warm through the night. Twenty-year-old first-time diplomat Bernard Boursicot is alone at the French embassy's Christmas party. Shi Pei Pu, on the other hand, is crowded by a horde of guests. All stand, heel-to-heel, glossy-eyed, hypnotized by the former opera singer's magnetism, by a persona that seems far larger than the man's petite physical stature.

Boursicot's curiosity grows with each sip of his cocktail and he waits until Shi is finally alone before approaching him. The twenty-year-old notices how alluring Shi is: delicate features, soft pillowy lips, doe eyes, and a dewy complexion that glows under the holiday lights. Shi is in his mid-twenties but could easily pass as much younger, awkwardly sporting a Mao-style suit that cloaks him, a little too large. He seems fragile against Boursicot, who towers over him at five feet nine. By the end of the night, Boursicot asks for Shi's contact details. He will regret this night for the rest of his life.

The next few weeks are a breathtaking whirlwind of dates around the city. As the two become close, Shi opens up about his past as a performer.

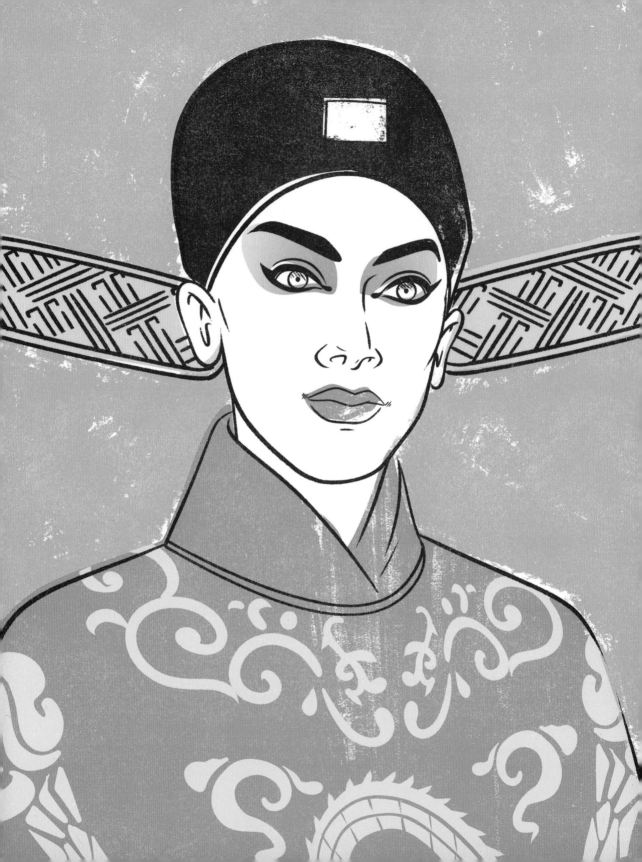

One of his most pivotal roles was in one of the most famous Chinese opera *The Story of the Butterfly,* in which Shi played the role of a beautiful girl who dons her brother's clothes in order to attend school, which only boys were allowed to do. There, she falls in love with another student. At first, the boy is confused—homosexuality is illegal. When he discovers that she's a woman, he asks her for hand in marriage. But it's too late, she's already betrothed to another man, and her family forces her to move away. The opera ends with the man dying of heartache and the girl succumbing to her own death on top of his tomb—only to be turned into butterflies. Little did Boursicot know that the play would foreshadow events to come in their own lives.

The role made Shi a local celebrity. Only men could participate in Chinese opera at the time, which meant the most beautiful men were cast in female roles. And Shi was gorgeous. Photos of him onstage are nothing short of awe-inspiring; he wears an ornate headpiece and a majestic dress, his face painted white and his cheekbones contoured so sharply, they could cut peach blossoms in half. Creamy crimson spills from his eyelids onto his cheeks and lips. His eyebrows are dark, symmetrically painted in, as is the perfect winged cat's-eye eyeliner, in strokes that called to mind calligraphy.

Months later, Boursicot decides to leave China permanently. When he invites Shi to his home for the first time to break the news, Shi confesses: "That story of the butterfly—it is my story, too." Shi explains that he had been forced to live as a boy after his mother gave birth to two girls and was threatened with replacement unless she bore a son for the family. Until now he—no, she—had been living a lie. Shi pleads with the Frenchman to swear to keep this a secret.

The news changes everything. Boursicot had been seeking a wife all these years, and Shi's announcement seems like fate. Boursicot had messed around with boys in high school, but his goal had always been to start a "traditional" family, though he'd never actually been with a woman. Attracted to Shi from the start, it seems right that they consummate their relationship. It's Boursicot's first time with a woman, and he's nervous. He doesn't know if he'll be any good. He's ignorant of the contours of a woman's body, not aware of every detail of their curves. When they finally make love, thrusting their bodies together, Boursicot realizes there's no passion at all. The sex is clumsy. In future encounters, the lights are always turned off and Shi always takes full control, often forbidding Boursicot to look at her body. "Let me do it," Shi would demand every time. Boursicot doesn't give it much thought, assuming that all Chinese women are modest when it comes to their approach in the bedroom and that this is normal.

A few weeks pass and Shi says she's pregnant. "If it's a boy, name him Bertrand," Boursicot says on his way to the airport, off to explore other parts of the world.

He returns to China four years later, having found another job with the French embassy in Beijing. Still thinking about Shi, he contacts her, and when they meet he discovers he's the father of a square-faced boy, Bertrand Shi Du Du, who looks nothing like him. He and Shi are now allowed to meet freely, as she's been assigned as his Chinese tutor. A few months later, she's replaced with a government official named Kang. Boursicot doesn't think much of it and is grateful that Kang allows him to continue meeting with his lover. In the coming months, the two become good friends. When Kang requests French government documents, Boursicot has no qualms about handing them over. They're useless, he thinks. By the time he returns to Paris, he's given over thousands of classified forms.

After Boursicot leaves China for good, he finds a way to bring both Shi and the child to him to Paris in 1982 after finagling a three-month cultural visa for Shi to lecture about China. When the two arrive, Shi becomes a sensation. Requests for her to perform come flooding in. Shi extends her stay, booking shows and delighting Parisians with her extravagant stage gowns, perfectly painted face, and dazzling presence. A year passes, and she and Bertrand have created a life together—they've made friends, and outside of China, Shi can finally live freely as a woman.

Little do they know, they're being trailed by agents from the Direction de la Surveillance du Territoire, the French domestic intelligence service, who are curious about Shi's relationship with Boursicot. Boursicot is brought in for questioning, then arrested on charges of espionage; they have a decade's worth of evidence from Boursicot's diplomatic work in China and his close relationship with Kang. In the matter of a week, Boursicot is thrown into Fresnes, a men's prison—and is outraged when he discovers that his lover has been thrown in with him, also on espionage charges. It's unsafe for a woman to be here, he complains. He receives the truth in his cell, while listening to a radio announcer reporting on the justice ministry's medical findings. "The Chinese Mata Hari, who was accused of spying, is a man!"

A man.

In a courtroom only six months later, Shi and Boursicot stand beside each other. Boursicot wears a suit with a striped tie, his hands behind his back. The Chinese performer sports an oversize black blazer, hair neatly parted. Both look defeated as they retell their love story. The Christmas party, how they dated in the shadows. Shi even divulges details about the first time they have sex.

"I never told Bernard I was a woman," Shi claims. "I only let it be understood that I could be a woman." Boursicot is disgusted as he can't believe what he's hearing. It's later revealed that Shi purchased a biracial baby from a Uighur doctor and passed him off as Boursicot's own. But Shi will not admit guilt, nor that they had intended to destroy Boursicot personally or politically. Later, Shi would say this about their identity: "I thought France was a democratic country, is it important if I am a man or a woman?" We may never be able to confirm Shi's understanding of self—man, woman, or nonbinary.

Months later, Shi would receive a French presidential pardon, to avoid straining relations between France and the already embarrassed Chinese government. Boursicot would be pardoned four months later, after investigators discover nothing of importance among the documents he had handed over to Kang. "If this case is anything, it is a crime of passion," the defense would argue.

Shi would never go back to the country that had so limited their expression of self, and would continue performing as an opera singer in France until the end of their life. Shi and Boursicot would speak infrequently through the years. Boursicot would end up in a nursing home in his later years, lonelier than ever. In 2009, months before Shi passed, they called Boursicot, revealing that even after all these years, the deception, the trials, the heartache, they still loved him. It would be the last time they'd ever speak.

(CHAPPED) LIPS DON'T LIE

Say goodbye to chapped lips forever.

Whether or not you're in the mood for love, use this quick guide to get supple, hydrated, healthy—and kissable—lips!

Lipsmack. There are a mul-titude of reasons why your lips are chapped. For one, they have no sweat glands and fewer oil glands, which is one reason there are so many natural wrinkles to them. They only get drier with each gust of hot air you expel, in places with low humidity, and when exposed to extremely cold or heat. And when you add saliva to the equation . . . just know that each smack, lick, and bite will dry your lips out further.

Scrub-a-Dub. If your lips are seriously chapped, try a lip scrub. These usually include sugar crystals that naturally slough off dead skin cells. You can also mix honey and granulated sugar together for an amazingly effective DIY scrub.

Slick and Slide. For your lips to become happy and healthy, they need products that are a humectant *and* occlusive. The former is a fancy word for any ingredient that brings in moisture and the latter for sealing it shut. Petroleum jelly is a popular occlusives, but those who want cleaner ingredients can look for shea, mango, and cocoa butters and unrefined coconut oil. Humectants can be found in ingredients like glycerin, honey, and hyaluronic acids.

Sleep It Off. They say you lose a lot of moisture at night while your skin tries to repair itself. This goes for your lips as well. To wake up with the softest lips, try a lip mask. It's thicker than a lip balm and prevents any moisture from evaporating during the night.

Humidify! If you live in a dry climate, or during the colder winter months, use a humidifier. It will keep your skin overall, nose, and throat happy and healthy as well.

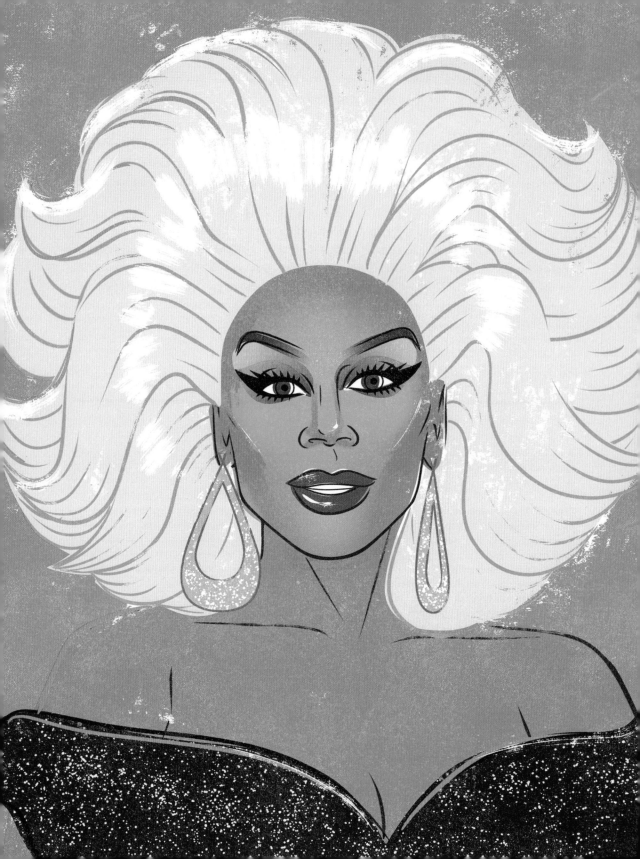

RUPAUL

(1 9 6 0 -)

The Queen of Queens.

"DRAG IS DANGEROUS," RUPAUL ANDRE CHARLES, THE MOTHER of drag, once said to the *Hollywood Reporter.* "Drag is not politically correct. Drag will never be mainstream." Of course, *RuPaul's Drag Race* defied *all* expectations—even his own—strutting into the herstory books as one of the biggest reality shows ever. Earning RuPaul four consecutive Emmys for best host, the multi-season series not only became an international sensation—over ninety-one countries have licensed it for syndication—but put drag on the pop culture map.

For those living under a rock, *Drag Race* is a weekly reality show that brings a diverse roster of queens to *serve* looks, *beat* faces, and *snatch* wigs, in hopes of becoming America's next drag superstar. *Drag Race* is all about beauty, humor, stage presence, costumes, couture, and lots and lots of drama. What's so remarkable about the show isn't the competition, but its ability to be authentic to its community. It's always been *for* LGBTQIA *by* LGBTQIA. The show aired on the Logo channel for eight seasons before making the move to VH1, providing an even bigger platform for all to enjoy the uplifting nature of drag culture.

After three decades strutting his stuff and getting glammed from head to toe everywhere from nightclubs to television screens, RuPaul is finally getting the recognition he deserves. But getting there was far from easy. For a drag queen to get respect took not only tenacity and hard work but also charisma, uniqueness, nerve, and talent.

RuPaul's stardom didn't come by accident. When a psychic told Ernestine Fontinette that her son was going to be world-famous, she had no doubt that he'd become a star. The year was 1960, and Ernestine, who went by Toni, already had two seven-year-old girls, a set of twins named Renette and Renae. Her husband, Irving Charles, was an electrician. Both had relocated to California from the Deep South during the period we now know as the Great Migration. Before her baby was born, she came up with a name: Roux, she'd decided, as in the essential flour-and-butter base used for dishes like étouffée and jambalaya, a nod to her Louisiana heritage.

She would eventually shorten Roux to "Ru" and added "Paul," and when RuPaul Andre Charles finally arrived, Toni knew his unique moniker would make him famous. "Ain't another motherfucker alive with a name like that," she said. In the Charles household, RuPaul grew up as the center of attention. It wasn't only because he was a boy. The prettiest one out of the four children (his mother would eventually have a fourth and final child, Rozy), he had an effervescent personality that always seemed too large for his frame. All along, the entire family knew RuPaul was different—not just vibrant, fearless, and talented, but also gay.

Over the years, his childhood became more unstable as Toni and Irving's relationship became tumultuous. Things got so heated one day that Toni doused Irving's car with gasoline and threatened to throw a book of matches onto it. RuPaul knew it was time to escape, and he ended up moving to Atlanta to live with his older sister. There he attended a performance arts school where he could channel his creative energy. But school wasn't for him, and he quit soon after he'd enrolled, instead getting a job selling used cars to get by.

This wasn't how he'd imagined his life would be. RuPaul was destined to be an internation- ally recognized name—the psychic had said it, his mother had believed it. Convinced by his destiny, RuPaul moved to New York City to seek his destiny. There, he became a go-go dancer at the Pyramid Club. Though he found some success, it wasn't until he threw on a wig, sissied his walk, and shantayed onstage that he became a sought-after nightclub fix- ture. It only helped that his 6-foot-4-inch stature was elevated to over 7 feet by heels and a larger-than-life blond wig. Soon, he became a local icon in the downtown scene, being photographed with the hottest club kids, suddenly a celebrity among the rebellious young twentysomethings. But for all his popularity, he was broke—and superstardom still seemed to be a farfetched idea.

"Nothing was clicking," he later recalled to the *Guardian*. "It was my Saturn returns, and it was that crossroads. I wasn't sure if the prophet was true." He was contemplating suicide, about to give it all up, when Oprah came on screen. On her daytime talk show, the media mogul spoke to him through the television as if she was the oracle herself: "Don't you dare give up."

While New York City loved him, mainstream culture was afraid of his gender expression. A man in drag wasn't only unusual in the 1980s, it was perceived as wicked by America's Christian standards. As much as RuPaul wanted to break through to the mainstream, it seemed as if America wasn't ready. Would it ever be?

But he was undeterred. In between perfecting his drag persona—from his humor to his stage presence—he was creating magic in the background. By night, he was a larger-than-life performer, but by day, he was busy writing and recording a secret demo tape. He decided music was the only way he could reach the masses and become mainstream. He recorded a demo for a track called "Supermodel (You Better Work)" and sent it to Tommy Boy Records. They signed him immediately. In 1992, the song became an international smash hit, topping the charts. "Work! Turn to the left. Work! Now turn to the right! Work! Sashay, shantay."

His plan for domination had worked. Not only did the song top the charts, it put RuPaul at the center of the national consciousness. He made appearances on *The Arsenio Hall Show* in 1993, becoming the first drag queen to guest on a late-night show. The historic moment not only showcased RuPaul's glamour, but bewitched audiences around the world who had no other choice but to fall in love with the young star. Next would come his first cosmetics campaign with MAC Cosmetics, where he was the brand's first-ever drag spokesperson. In 1996 VH1 greenlit his talk show, *The RuPaul Show,* making history again as the first-ever openly gay person to host a talk show. With guests ranging from Diana Ross to Cher, the show would go on for one hundred episodes before being canceled.

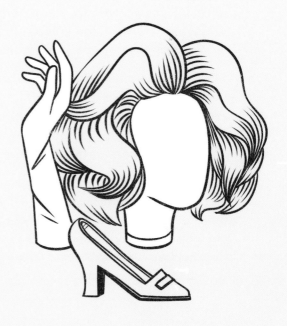

At the end of 1998, RuPaul began to look within to find what the universe was really telling him. Was his career over? Was this the end of drag? It seemed as if all signs were pointing to yes. It almost seemed as if the world was becoming more conservative than ever. There were no openly gay characters on television, let alone drag queens. While retiring the wig, RuPaul embraced self-care and self-love, exercising, therapy, and delving into what he was *really* passionate about.

After a decade under the radar, away from Hollywood, RuPaul felt he was finally ready. The political climate had changed under Barack Obama, and it felt like the perfect time to make a comeback. He was ready to sashay back onto screens with a vengeance. And in 2009, he did just that, ideating a show called *RuPaul's Drag Race.* The show was pitched to multiple networks but was rejected for being "too niche" (a euphemism for "too homosexual"). Finally, it found a home on Logo, an LGBTQIA network under Viacom, where it was given the greenlight for a couple of seasons.

But RuPaul wasn't playing around. He had big dreams for drag culture. It wasn't *just* for the gays, either—he wanted drag to go mainstream. The reality show's sticky concept was in its format: every week, drag contestants would compete in weekly tasks, strutting their stuff, primping their wigs, while reading for filth. While the drama was entertaining and the outfits over the top, what really made the show remarkable were the human stories of resilience, coming to terms with identity, and authenticity. It didn't hurt that the show handpicked a diverse and inclusive roster of contestants who represented several underrepresented communities not usually visible in the mainstream media.

Overnight, RuPaul resurrected his career. And in time, he became an even bigger star than he'd been in the '90s. Eight years later, in 2017, the show was picked up by VH1, where its viewership doubled. It would pick up multiple Emmys and other awards, earning recognition as the top show on television and making history as the most successful LGBTQIA show ever. The bigger impact was that drag was no longer an underground form of entertainment.

Needless to say, Toni's psychic was right all along. RuPaul not only became a worldwide celebrity, but *the* most famous drag star in all of herstory. On the set of season 6, RuPaul sported a powder pastel suit, which looked ever so chicly shrunken on his 6-foot-4 frame. As he did every season, Mama Ru had a mantra stitched on the inside collar of his shirt. "You're born naked," it read in bold letters. "And the rest is drag."

"YOU'RE BORN NAKED, and THE REST IS DRAG."

— RUPAUL

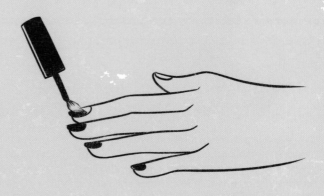

A Drag Starter Kit from the biggest fish herself, Plastique Tiara.

When it comes to drag, the fishier, the better. Well, at least according to *RuPaul's Drag Race* season 11 contestant Plastique Tiara. (For those who don't know what "fish" means, the fishier you are, the more convincing you are as a cisgender woman.) For Plastique Tiara—who's amassed millions of followers thanks to her dramatic transformations and is perhaps "the" drag queen of TikTok—becoming a fishy queen hasn't been easy.

"I never felt beautiful growing up," she says. Born in Vietnam as Duc Tran Nguyen, Plastique Tiara immigrated to Dallas as a child. "Not only was I that quiet kid who didn't understand anything in school, but chubby and with bad acne." All that changed when Nguyen watched *RuPaul's Drag Race* in high school. "I finally felt like I found people who had the same interests as me!"

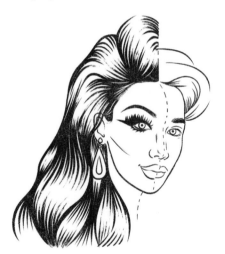

Nguyen was living a *Hannah Montana* life, secretly putting on makeup for fun, then wiping it away before coming back home. When his mother finally saw him in makeup, she gasped. "She was afraid that somehow [being] a guy in makeup would bring even more negative attention towards me, and wasn't approving at first," he says. But after a couple of weeks, she came around to the idea. Today, she's one of Plastique Tiara's biggest supporters.

"You only gain confidence through time," Nguyen says. "Looking back, I looked busted as fuck, but you have to think that you're beautiful inside and that you'll turn the party no matter what. Being different brings you opportunities, and your own uniqueness is amazing."

Here Nguyen breaks down every single product and tool to get the *fishiest* drag makeup. "It's all about technique, which you'll find on your own—you don't need all of these products, for instance," Nguyen says. "But more makeup will only help. Yes, more is more!"

Now let's go fish!

EYES

Lashes: "Go to the local beauty supply store, skip places like Sephora—it's not gonna cut it," Plastique says. The lashes there are too short. If you're starting out with drag, you'll want at least 20-millimeter lashes or up to 25 millimeters. "Stack your lashes—always."

Lash curler: "I used to curl my eyelashes with a spoon because I was broke, now [I use a curler by] Shiseido, which is really great for my personal eye shape."

Mascara: Waterproof all day, every day. Especially in drag and performance. For this, Plastique goes for two separate products. "Honestly, I love all drugstore products, like L'Oréal Voluminous, which would be the only things I could afford when I was younger. I like MAC Extended Play for the bottom lashes because the brush is really tiny."

Color contacts: "When I want that pop, I go with Desio, but these days, I don't even wear contacts. I'm going for the natural look." (For non-prescription lenses, make sure to read the safety on brand sites, including but not limited to its FAQs, safety testing, and rule and regulations it abides by. Safety, friends, is key!)

Undereye powder: Plastique uses MAC Studio Fix. "It's great for undereyes and everywhere to bake." (See page 22 for more on baking.)

Highlight: "Rather than contouring so much," Plastique says, "I only use a highlight for my nose and literally will paint on an exclamation point down, down to the dot. It's not as harsh."

Eyeshadow: "I'd invest in a good foundation and eyeshadows—everything else can be whatever. Eyeshadow from KimChi Chic Beauty are so pigmented and really go a long way."

FACE

Color Corrector: Plastique's go-to is Cover FX in Orange, but, she says, "If you're on a budget, L.A. Girl has a good one, too." Color correcting is essential in drag makeup: "I luckily don't have a lot of facial hair, thank God! But Orange is great for canceling out the blue tint that's left over from shaving and shows through in drag."

Foundation: "MAC Full Coverage is the only product that works for my sensitive skin." To find the right shade, Plastique recommends spending a long time at a makeup counter. If that's not possible, some beauty brands can match your color online and send you a couple of shades to test before you buy. Taking the time to test out several products also allows you to discover if certain ingredients do not work well with your skin. "For me, it's silicone—I can't use that ingredient. It actually breaks me out, but I found this at eighteen only through testing."

Bronzer: "I'll use a darker shade from Anastasia Beverly Hills to contour, along with the lighter shade from Marc Jacobs."

Bake: Powder (Plastique uses Coty) to allow the makeup to stay.

Blush: Plastique uses MAC Cosmetics Love Me Blush for her signature look.

Setting Spray: A product that preserves your makeup for longer wear and prevents smudging. "Morphe's is only like, $10, but it's great as a last step. But also if you go overboard with the powder, this will help."

BROWS

Kryolan TV Paint Stick: Drag makeup is all about painting in brows, a reason why many drag queens shave theirs. For those who want to keep their brows, stick glue is a must. "It's a staple to really block out all of the brows. This product—it really does hide everything."

Brow powder and pomade: "The Anastasia Beverly Hills fills in realistic brows and comes in a variety of shades. I still have so much of this product left over from my time on *RuPaul.*"

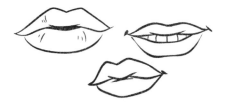

LIPS

Lip liner: "Morphe's [Color Pencil in] 'Bite Me' is very affordable and under $4."

Lipstick: "I love KimChi Chic Beauty's Natural shade, it's my go-to. The lip gloss as well is so good."

FINAL TOUCH

Confidence: "You gain confidence from time, but you need that initial push into makeup. I didn't know what I'd look like in drag, but you have to experiment, think of that illusion and go for it. That's what drag's all about—turning it out and creating a world you want. That's power right there."

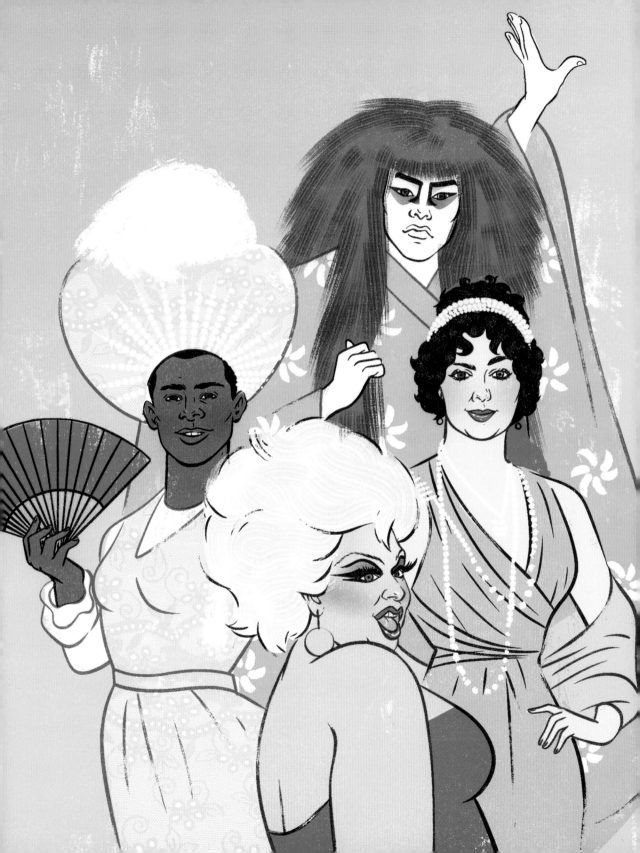

DRAG QUEENS: A HERSTORY

They came, they strutted, they slayed.

OF COURSE, *RuPaul's Drag Race* didn't discover drag culture. It did, however, begin to normalize it. Drag is an art form that has been alive and vibrant for centuries in multiple countries around the world. At its core, drag has always been about transgressive power, rebellion against societal norms, fighting against the patriarchy by playing with gender roles with lipstick, powder, and a big wig. But like RuPaul once said, "Drag is there to remind culture not to take itself so seriously. All of this is illusion."

In Japan during the Edo period (1603–1868), Kabuki was becoming popular thanks to a woman named Izumo no Okuni. She created an entirely new genre of dramatic entertainment with a troupe of female performers, who played characters of both sexes. They would become so in-demand that they were requested by the Imperial Court—but in an all too familiar narrative, they were eventually shut down by the government, ostensibly for being too erotic. They would be replaced by men, known as *yaro-kabuki,* who played both male and female roles and quickly rose to popularity. It was during this period where the art of Kabuki became even more elaborate. Kumadori, the stage makeup for Kabuki men became standardized and an art form all performers were required to study. Makeup was worn in symmetrical patterns, and colors were essential in performance, as they indicated the actor's part. Red signified the hero, while blue represented the villain. Brown was used for spirits and monsters, usually demons. Lips were also essential in describing who an actor was. For instance, painting an actor's lips with a thicker bottom lip showed femininity; corners painted downward signified a noble character. The art of Kabuki is still practiced today, and is the most popular traditional style of Japanese drama.

The word "drag" is thought to have originated in the late sixteenth century, during Shakespeare's time, when only men were allowed to perform onstage. This meant that female characters were played by men wearing makeup, wigs, and long dresses that would *drag* across the floor. In the 1700s drag masquerades boomed in popularity, taking place in brothels, theaters, public gardens, and assembly rooms. One party called Midnight Masquerades reportedly drew a crowd of 800 people a week. Looks thrown together included men who dressed themselves like nursing maids, witches, and bawds (women who managed brothels), among others.

One of the first drag queens during this time was a man named John Cooper, who went by his drag name, Princess Seraphina. A regular at underground gay bars, she was given respect and never encountered harassment from the local authorities. The only scandal she's said to have been involved in was when she was assaulted by men who stole her clothing and jewelry.

In 1870 "drag" became an official term to describe men dressed as women. In a British newspaper, a cheeky invitation wrote that a man was "having a musical party he thought he would make it a little fancy dress affair." It went on to say: "We shall come in drag, which means men wearing women's costumes."

Drag culture thrived in British underground cultures, often hidden from the mainstream and the police. When word got out that London was a hub for such parties and gatherings, police targeted any man they thought carried a hint of suspicion. To be gay in England during this time was criminal. Raids on drag gatherings were carried out into the 1930s, and more than one man caught in attendance was thrown into prison.

In the US, the first drag queen to self-identify as such was a man named William Dorsey Swann, whose friends called him "the Queen." Swann, who had formerly been enslaved, became legendary for throwing extravagant soirees known as drag balls in the Washington, D.C. area. The gatherings were held in secret at places like the local YMCA, which had guests wearing silk dresses, corsets, bustles, long hose, and slippers, "everything that goes to make a female's dress complete," said one report from the *Washington Critic*. Some of Swann's looks included a corseted pink satin dress, a gigantic wig, false diamond earrings, pearl necklaces, long pantyhose, and slippers. "It was very gaudy," says historian Channing Joseph. Swann's parties often included a competition called a Cakewalk (a now racist term, after its appropriation by white minstrels), where former enslaved drag queens mimicked the gestures of pretentious masters and mistresses. "They'd cock their heads back in an aristocratic manner, flick their wrists downwards, lean back in an exaggerated walk and improvise around a theme or category, twisting and turning back," Joseph says. Whoever won would receive a cake as the prize. These underground drag balls continued to be held for years, until Swann was outed by the media. In his later years, Swann took up sewing and tailoring but would move back in with his parents. He's said to have died alone on Christmas Day 1925, and no one came to claim his body. But his spirit of drag would live on in another generation.

In the 1920s and 1930s, hundreds gathered at the Hamilton Lodge in Harlem, a space for Black queer people, called "fairies" for being feminine and dressing in drag. These parties soon became the most popular nightlife spot in the East Coast, if not in the entire country. "The masculine women and feminine men, how are you going to tell the roosters from the hens?" One ball event in 1929 got so big, over 2,000 people were turned away. These "fag-gots balls" became the hottest tickets in town. As reported in the *New York Age* in 1926, the parties were attended by up to 1,500 people, half of whom were wearing "gorgeous evening gowns, wigs and powdered faces . . . hard to distinguish from many of the women."

Soon, drag became mainstream entertainment throughout America thanks to a man named Julian Eltinge. Long before RuPaul made her debut with the Club Kids of the '90s, Eltinge was heating up Broadway and Hollywood with his remarkable ability to transform into a woman with a high-fashion sensibility. As a child he'd appeared in the Boston Cadets Revue and debuted in women's clothing at ten years old. By the time he became a young adult, he'd perfected his feminine voice, makeup, and hair, and had appeared in vaudeville per-formances. His drag look was so convincing, audiences weren't sure if Eltinge was male or female. To puzzle them, he toured under his first name and went by his last in his day-to-day life. The schtick that never seemed to fail was taking off his wig and makeup at the end of each performance, revealing his true identity to the stunned crowd. While Eltinge perfected femininity, offstage he had to perform masculinity with hypermachoism. At the time, drag performance wasn't necessarily linked to the LGBTQIA community, and as such, Eltinge fought against "homosexual panic," ensuring that to the outside world, he was completely, utterly, unquestionably straight.

However, by the mid-1900s, the jig was up: the LGBTQIA community no longer wanted to confine their identity expressions to the night, or to the stage. Binaries were not codified in laws that prohibited people who appeared in a "dress not belonging to their sex," like a 1954 law passed in Denver. In 1959, an LA law stated that if a person's gender presentation did not match their ID card, they would be thrown in prison. This enraged the LGBTQIA community. In one of the first queer uprisings in American history, called the Cooper Do-nuts riots, drag queens, transgender women, gay men, and lesbian women in Los Angeles united against the police. A couple of years later in San Francisco, drag queens stood by their transgender friends in the Compton's Cafeteria riot, after police were called on transgender individuals. In New York City, drag queens and transgender women were at the forefront of the Stonewall riots, protesting the law, demanding equal rights for their communities.

Two decades later in 1984, LGBTQIA arrests had decreased (though "walking while trans" laws still existed, and do even in the present), and drag was celebrated in a more public setting with Wigstock, an annual event held in New York's Tompkins Square Park and later in Union Square. The annual outdoor event brought together several drag performers, including Divine, a 300-pound queen who was allegedly the muse for Ursula, the villain in Disney's *The Little Mermaid.* The event was the first time that drag queens could be visible in public spaces and revel with LGBTQIA and non-LGBTQIA people alike. In the late 1980s and 1990s, drag became commonplace in New York's queer clubs, thanks to downtown culture. The Club Kids ushered in a newfound freedom of expression. Uptown, drag balls were having a moment, with houses of mostly Black and Latinx community members holding competitions for different categories of "walks" and for vogueing, a camp dance named after the fashion magazine.

Drag culture would meet the mainstream again with the launch of *The RuPaul Show,* a nationally syndicated talk show, and then again a decade later with the debut of *RuPaul's Drag Race* in 2009. Through every era, while costumes may have changed, the spirit of drag has stayed the same: it has always been about seeking freedom of expression and joy. It has been entertainment, whether as formal art like the Japanese kabuki or for private parties like Swann's.

The same spirit lives on in our current age. Today, drag is celebrated as an art form by people from young to old. Drag is all about love, acceptance, and transgression, but above all else, fun. We now are witnessing drag queens taking over Instagram, becoming the face of brands ranging from beverages to cosmetics, and becoming actors in their own right. And they're more diverse than ever, with performers ranging from androgynous to "fishy" (aka extremely feminine or cisgender-female-passing) to goth, pageant, cosplay/anime, high fashion—and far beyond. It's remarkable to realize just how much the drag community has overcome and how resilient drag queens have been for so long. Finally, the queens are claiming their rightful thrones, basking in the spotlight, and ruling the world. As any queen would observe, it's all *sickening.*

AT ITS CORE, DRAG HAS ALWAYS BEEN ABOUT TRANSGRESSIVE POWER, REBELLION AGAINST SOCIETAL NORMS, FIGHTING AGAINST the PATRIARCHY by PLAYING with GENDER ROLES with LIPSTICK, POWDER, and A BIG WIG.

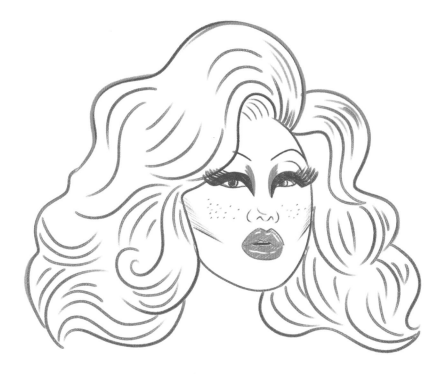

With the launch of KimChi Chic Beauty alongside NYX Cosmetics founder Toni Ko—who sold NYX to L'Oréal and then created her new brand, Bespoke Beauty Brands—*RuPaul's Drag Race* star Kim Chi has taken her love of makeup and channeled it into a burgeoning business. Here's how this world-renowned performer and beauty star does it all, without a smudge to her makeup.

First of all, how did you come up with your incredible drag name?

Kimchi is the national dish of Korea. I wanted a name that represents my culture but sounds feminine at the same time. Kim Chi seemed like the most natural fit!

Totally makes sense. As a Korean American, how was your experience doing drag in a city like Chicago?

I lived in Chicago for eleven years, all of my twenties. Chicago is a great place for emerging artists to experience the city life at a low living cost comparatively to other major cities. Chicago drag audiences celebrate all things weird and fun—as long as it's polished. Working in that sort of environment while working alongside many queens who are also regarded as legends now has helped and honed my craft. I wouldn't trade that experience for anything in the world!

Speaking of being polished, your makeup is known for being extremely editorial and next-level. Were you professionally trained?

It's all self-taught. A friend has helped me with the basics in the very beginning but from that point on, it was a lot of trial and error till I got to where I'm at today. Practice makes perfect, I suppose, though I'm far from perfect.

You're so confident with your performances onstage, and so fearless. How did your traditional Korean parents react to this?

It's almost every Asian American's struggle to live up to their family's expectation and wanting not to disappoint their parents. I realized, though, at the end of the day, I have to live my life for me, and only I can truly make myself happy and fulfilled.

What advice can you give to other young people who also want to live their truths?

Financial stability. It's not easy for everyone to achieve right away, but when you don't have to rely on anyone else to live, that's when you can truly make decisions to do things that make you happy.

We obviously need to talk about beauty. If someone was making a makeup starter kit, what essentials would they need?

Starting makeup is not a cheap thing. A good full-coverage foundation, a true black

eyeliner, pigmented lipstick with great formula is a must in anyone's kit. Also, a great set of lashes that suit your eye shape and makeup the best is a necessity!

So how does one find their most flattering makeup look?

Trial and error. Experiment and have fun. You never know if you feel your fantasy in hot pink eyeshadow until you try it and see yourself with it. It's all muscle memory, just like painting. The first few times will be a struggle and your hands will be shaky. The more you do it, the easier it'll be to create smooth lines and blending. Practice, practice, practice. You'll know you're doing it right the first time you achieve the perfect eyeliner.

Off to practice, as we speak! But before we go, what's left for Kim Chi to accomplish?

The past few years, I've been lucky and blessed enough to travel the world! Five continents, hundreds of cities, and back multiple times in a lot of the cities as well. For the future, I think I would like to work on myself, my brand and growing KimChi Chic Beauty on a global scale.

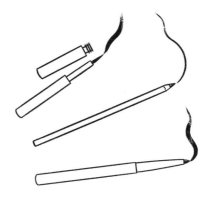

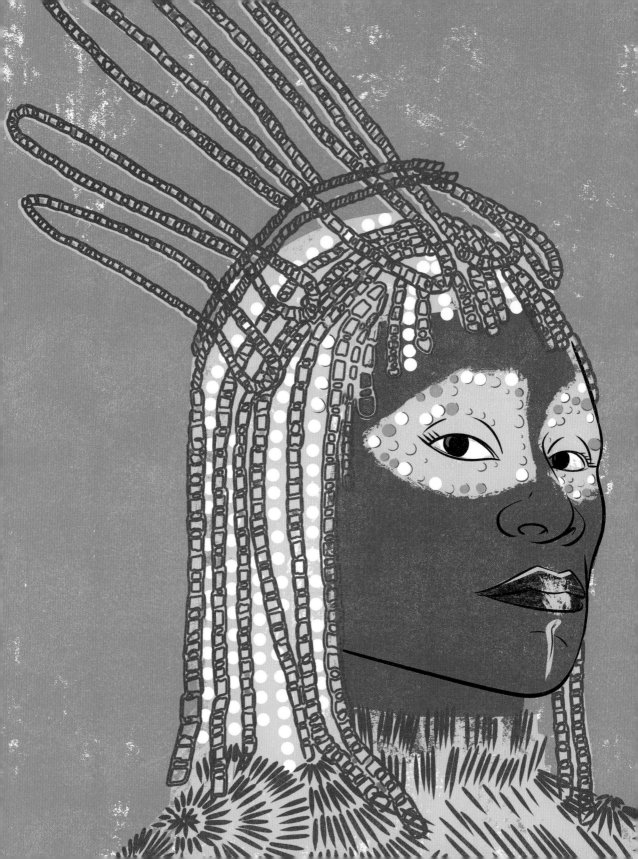

BILLY PORTER

(1 9 6 9 -)

The King of the Ball.

HE ENTERED ON A LITTER CARRIED BY SIX MEN IN GOLD CHAIN mail. Set down gently by his footmen, the sun god surveyed his kingdom in all his finery. Dripping in gold, he radiated fire, his 24-karat gold headpiece and jeweled catsuit glinting and catching in the light.

The light of the paparazzi's flashbulbs, that is. This isn't ancient Egypt (but see page 25 for more on that)—this was the 2019 Met Gala, where Billy Porter reigned over all.

This wasn't Billy's first rodeo—even if it was his first Met Gala! His beauty looks have always been here to slay. He was the belle of the ball during Saks Fifth Avenue's New York Fashion Week event, where he sported a fierce red-winged eye. At the 2020 Grammys, he wore a showstopping wide-brimmed turquoise hat, paired with matching eyeshadow. A few months before, at the Oscars, Billy waltzed down the red carpet in a tailored tuxedo jacket and velvet ball gown from Christian Siriano. His dress clearly won the night—and wearing 5-inch heels, Billy stomped all over the tired tropes of traditional masculinity, the stale messages about male celebrities and what they should look like. Of course, Billy wasn't about beauty just for beauty's sake. At the Tony Awards, Billy wore a red-and-pink velvet suit with a uterus-shaped train encrusted in 30,000 Swarovski crystals in support of women's right to choose. "I'm an advocate for all who are disenfranchised," he told the *Hollywood Reporter*. "None of us are free until we're all free!"

Billy's journey to glamour, glitz, and activism wasn't an easy one, though. Growing up as a gay Black boy in inner-city Pittsburgh, Billy was a target. He wasn't good at sports or faking machismo to fit in at school, and at home, his stepfather sexually abused Billy from age seven to twelve. Leaning into his talents of singing, dancing, and performing, he used everything he had to get out. At fifteen, he packed his bags, found a job as an amusement park performer, and sang and danced under the lights of the Tilt-a-Whirl, before making his way to Carnegie Mellon University, where he studied theater. At the ripe old age of twenty-one, Billy set his sights on Broadway and began booking parts. Lots of them. First came *Grease* and *Jesus Christ Superstar*. Then came a role in *Smokey Joe's Cafe* that impressed music executives from A&M Records so much that they signed him almost overnight.

But the deal came with a caveat: Billy would have to conform to the label's traditional standards of masculinity and "minimize" his gay, repressing his authentic self. This was the mid-nineties, after all, an era saturated with hypermasculinity and rampant misogyny. The biggest R&B hits of the time were R. Kelly's "Bump n' Grind" and Ginuwine's "Pony," both of which focused on using a woman's body for the sole sexual gratification of a man. The R&B stars of this era adopted lyrics about sexing up women, wore skin-baring clothing that showed off their hard bodies, and were about overt masculine performance. Men were expected to be overtly macho in their behavior, and chauvinism was a game that had to be won. It was a dark time in America for anyone who didn't publicly identify as straight. With the AIDS crisis still looming, and many spreading foul propaganda that HIV was "gay cancer," the public was fearful of the LGBTQIA community. To be gay in public meant that you were tainted, and labeled you as a risk for spreading disease.

"Don't open your mouth to talk," A&M execs instructed Billy. "[You're] too bubbly, people will know."

Billy's eponymous album dropped on his birthday, September 21, 1997, to rave reviews, but the trauma of being forced back into the closet was too much for him. A few months after the album's release, Billy marched into his CEO's office, quit on the spot, and left for Hollywood. But in Los Angeles, he encountered the same pushback. There just weren't roles for gay men on television, unless you counted the lone outlier of *Will & Grace*. And if you were black and gay? Forget about it.

Bankrupt and back in New York City, Billy finally had a spot of luck when he landed the part of Lola in *Kinky Boots.* It was on Broadway as Lola that Billy rediscovered his inner strength and what made him *him.* When the *Kinky Boots* writers tried to rewrite Lola—an effervescent, colorful character whose identity was rooted in being gay!—as straight, Billy dug his heels in. After all he'd been through, after all the rejection for being "too femme," the turmoil of being an openly gay actor, it was outrageous to think he'd play Lola as straight. His tenacity paid off and the producers caved, and Billy won his first Tony and Grammy Awards for his portrayal of Lola, both visibly out and proud.

These days, Billy stars as Pray Tell, the grandfather of all the legendary children of New York's ball culture, in FX's *Pose*—and perhaps finally playing a role onscreen that celebrates Black and brown queer culture has powered Billy's stunning, boundary-pushing red carpet appearances. At almost fifty, he has become one of Hollywood's hottest stars, landing *Vogue* interviews, *New York Times* profiles, and that coveted Met Gala invite from Anna Wintour. But remembering his own struggles, Billy continues to advocate for anyone who is disenfranchised, and he does it loud and proud, and with style. He's always been an advocate. It's just that now, the world is finally listening.

He's always been an advocate.
It's just that now,
the world is finally listening.

HOW TO GET THAT MAJESTIC GLOW

According to Beyoncé's makeup artist, Sir John.

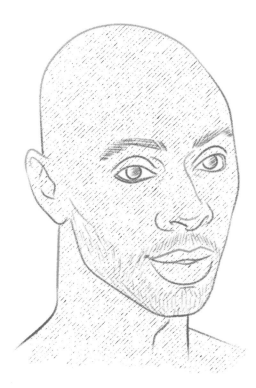

Behind Beyoncé's every move—from her multiple Met Gala appearances to that historic Coachella takeover—is Sir John, the genius responsible for her stunning *glow*. In between photoshoots, tours, and more, the beauty guru is also painting the world over with endorsement deals that take him from South Africa to Milan to New York City. Not only has Sir John become one of the most in-demand makeup artists of our time, he's creating his own empire.

The makeup artist, who also works with Naomi Campbell, Joan Smalls, and Viola Davis, among others, had to work all hours just to survive at first. He started as an assistant to the industry's top makeup artists including Pat McGrath and Charlotte Tilbury. Of course, being an assistant didn't pay the bills. In order to stay afloat, he'd run back to his apartment after work, take a short nap, then ride a subway to Queens, where he'd apply makeup to dancers at a strip club. On the dancers, he'd create over-the-top looks using bright pigments, golden shimmers, and blinding glitter. "That was extra because of how messy it was," he says in retrospect. "I had to charge at least $3 more for glitter." He worked two jobs for three entire years before he met Naomi Campbell at Milan Fashion Week, and then, of course, he met Beyoncé—and the rest is history.

Here Sir John takes us through his skincare regimen and describes how he gets his own—makeup-free or low-makeup!—glow on.

1. STARTS FROM WITHIN.

"It really does start from the gut," Sir John says. "If I have an event in a month and I want to look really dewy and great, I'll start taking probiotics. I'm so serious, they really do work." So do whole foods, like the antioxidant-rich blueberries, cleansing carrot juice, and celery, which detoxifies your kidneys. "You're purifying the body with these foods, and before you know it, your skin will be better."

PRO TIP: Skip the dairy. Sir John—along with many studies—says that dairy can increase your body's inflammatory response.

---

2. EXFOLIATION IS KEY . . .

Not everything is about applying makeup. For cosmetics to *really* work, you need a solid foundation. First things first: exfoliation. After cleansing, Sir John recommends chemical exfoliation in the form of acids like glycolic acid. "It will get rid of dead skin cells and allow your skin to breathe and reveal healthier skin naturally." Afterward, moisturize with a lotion, cream, or oil. "I especially like oils that also detoxify your pores and cleans them out," he says. Try oils rich with salicylic acids if you have acne, or with vitamin A, which promotes cell turnover. Or go for a lotion or cream moisturizer with another one of Sir John's favorite ingredients: "I love these serums and moisturizers with hyaluronic acid. Your body produces it naturally, but you need it topically to replenish what you've lost. Hyaluronic acids are powerful ingredients to get your skin to be super moisturized and healthy."

3. . . . SO IS MASSAGING YOUR FACE.

"The no-makeup look is honestly kind of what I'm doing right now for TV, which is basically great skincare habits and also, yes, massaging your face," he says. "That means break out your jade roller." If you don't have a jade roller, you can use your fingers or even a shot glass. "It's perfect for increasing circulation into your face." Circulation, Sir John says, is key. "You want to get the blood running or flowing to get that natural glow." Another hack to get your skin glowing from within is drinking a shot of beet juice an hour before your day begins. "It's great because it's a natural nitrate, so it opens up the blood vessels. But even taking a slight run can do wonders. Whenever you elevate your heart rate even for 30 minutes a day, it increases circulation." Then, it's all about using an SPF. "SPF gives you a natural glow just because of its ingredients. It's my go-to if I don't want to use any makeup." If SPF isn't giving you *enough* shine, try a non-shimmer highlighting stick or balm.

4. SCULPT IT OUT.

If you do want to use makeup, it's all about sculpting (aka chiseling out) the face, playing with shadow and light. Start with a foundation stick that's one shade deeper than your natural skin tone on specific areas of the face. This includes the sockets of your eyes, your cheekbones, jawline, anywhere that you find shadows. "Even a little bit of sculpting under the lash line will help!"

5. I CAN SEE YOUR HALO.

"What's glow? It's basically creating a halo of warmth around the face," Sir John says. "You want to mimic the sun when it's shining on you. Some parts are deeper in color, others are brighter." Sir John suggests tapping the high planes of the cheekbones, the center of the eyelids, and the line of the nose with a liquid or stick highlighter to balance out the shadows you've created with foundation.

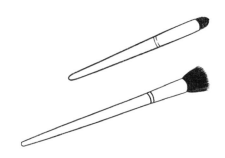

FRANK OCEAN'S BLOND(E) MOMENT

(1 9 8 7 -)

Individuality, sexuality, and duality.

THERE, ON THE COVER OF HIS SECOND STUDIO ALBUM, IS FRANK Ocean covering his eyes, a bandage wrapped around his forefinger. The image is tightly cropped, revealing a shower of light that reflects off his chiseled, sun-soaked body. His hair is dyed a sublime green. A cursory glance marks it as a beautiful portrait, but a closer examination reveals clues to a complex artist showing the world his desire to finally be *seen*. As an article in GQ would later describe, bleached hair has always represented rebellion. "In ancient Rome, prostitutes were required to dye their hair blond," the article explained. "Then the look spread to all levels of Roman society, as countercultural trends often do."

But the photograph wasn't the most confounding aspect of the album—it was the title. On the cover, "blond" is written in lowercase letters in a sans serif script. The word is italicized, bending to the right. But on music streaming sites, the title was changed, given an additional "e." When the album launched, Ocean uploaded a photo of himself on his infamous

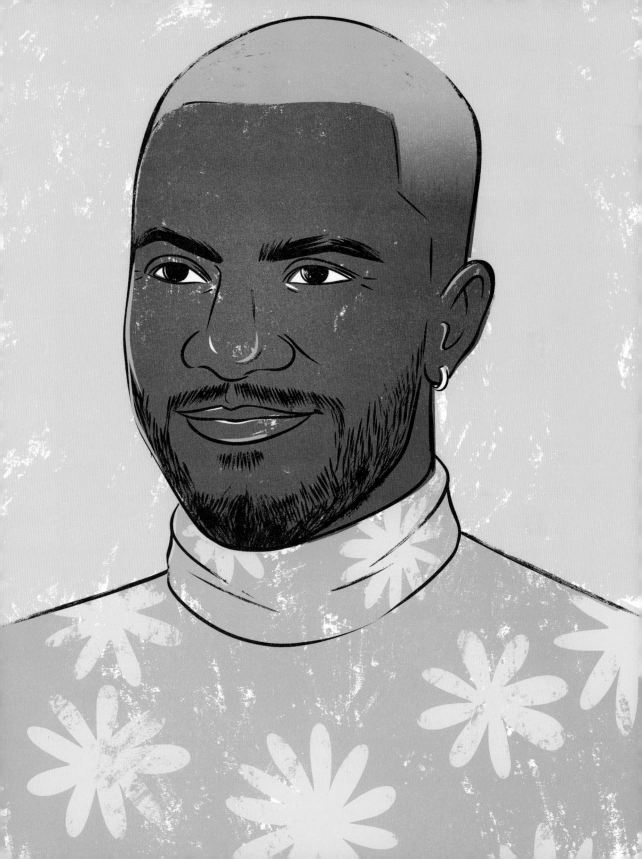

Tumblr, with the caption: ":) Birthday cake for Blonde." Had someone made a mistake on the album cover?

But this was Ocean, after all, wizard of inconspicuous meanings. The word "blond(e)" came into English from French. "Blonde" is a gendered noun for a woman with fair hair; its masculine equivalent is "blond." But "blond" as an adjective can be applied to anyone, of any gender. By using both spellings on and around his album, Ocean was playing with ambiguity, embracing duality.

This message is sprinkled throughout the album, which progresses where *channel Orange,* his first work, left off. *channel Orange* established Ocean as a music darling. But as the 62-minute masterpiece that is *blond(e)* gave small glimpses into his personal life, Ocean made history.

In a Tumblr post in cryptic capped letters, Frank Ocean came out in the most Frank Ocean way possible. "4 summers ago, I met somebody. I was 19. He was too," he wrote. "We spent that summer, and the summer after, together. Everyday almost. And on the days we were together, time would glide. I don't have any secrets I need to keep anymore . ?.?. I feel like a free man. I've never had more respect for life and living than I have right now." He would be one of the first R&B stars ever to do so.

The watershed event became sensational news, comparable to David Bowie's coming out in 1972 (see page 192 for more on Bowie). The 2010s were dominated by artists like Tyga, Chris Brown, and even Justin Bieber, who released popular songs celebrating hypermasculinity. To be outwardly queer in hip-hop and R&B was unthinkable, as there wasn't a single well-known queer artist to follow. Yet while Bowie may have encountered homophobia, Ocean's peers—from Jay-Z and Beyoncé to Tyler, The Creator and Russell Simmons—quickly lent their support. And with the drop of *blond(e),* Frank Ocean opened the floodgates of his creativity with an output of queer art.

Take the music video for the album's lead single, "Nike." The track is about youth, nostalgia, hedonism, buying Nikes. With high-pitched falsetto mixed with a lower chest voice, Ocean reckons with his younger self. In the five-minute video, we witness (in addition to a rapping chihuahua!) Ocean sporting beautiful wing eyeliner. Mesmerizing, dreamy, pure fantasy, the video glistens as vibrantly as the glitter on Ocean's face. It's almost a replica from Ocean's magazine, *Boys Don't Cry* (which debuted before the album), where he's photographed with eyeliner and silver eyeshadow that seems to paint his cheeks and speckle onto his beard.

Ocean's new expressive openness made him an instant beauty star. He started hair color trends, with the internet going wild over his millennial pink shade, his ICEE-blue ombré, and, of course, his different hues of green. When he dropped his skincare routine in 2019—"I need the night cream because when I wake up I feel very beautiful, moisturized, and ready to have people making eye contact with me, ready to look above my eyebrow, below the eyebrow. That's the life hack right there . . . you can't have the retinol in your creams in the day because it makes you more sun-sensitive, so you wanna throw that on at night"—it again went viral.

blond(e) was an alluring, compelling, and complex signal that a man could be beautiful, fluid, neither one nor the other, or both, with his identity as with anything else proving that perhaps blond(e)s really do have more fun. . . .

"I need the night cream because when I wake up I feel very beautiful, moisturized, and ready to have people making eye contact with me, ready to look above my eyebrow, below the eyebrow."

—FRANK OCEAN

HOW TO GET AN AT-HOME FACIAL

*Treat yourself to a spa-level experience—
in the comfort of your own bathroom.*

Want a glow-up without shelling out too much dough? Thankfully, you can take the products you already have in your medicine cabinet and massage yourself to a spa-grade facial. "People overcomplicate at-home facials," says NYC's premier aesthetician, Sofie Pavitt. "You really can get maximum results all by yourself." Here Sofie gives us a step-by-step guide to massaging your pores until your face gleams. All you need are your hands and a little bit of product. Let's go!

1. CLEANSE, EXFOLIATE, TREAT, REPEAT.

The three basic components of a facial? You're probably already doing them: cleansing your pores, exfoliating to remove any dead skin cells, and then treating with a serum. The last step is key, Sofie says, as your skin is usually depleted of vitamins and nutrients by the end of the day. Whether you're using a serum with vitamin C for brightening, hyaluronic acid for plumping and hydration, or peptides to build collagen, even a little can do a lot. "You've already done half the work by using a serum because it instantly sinks into the skin," she says. Finally, adding a sheet mask will give you all the benefits of your serums while locking hydration into your skin.

2. TONE UP.

If you want a massage, apply your moisturizers, serums, and oils with an upward motion. "You're fighting gravity all the way by doing this," Sofie says. Take your fingers and gently push your skin upward, starting from your chin and moving upward into the jawline. You can then stop at your temporomandibular joint (aka TMJ) and massage the tension. Repeat this a few times to not only release stress in your face but also drain any excess fluid into the lymphatic system. "Just make sure you're not pulling it. You don't want to be super aggressive with your motions." While there's no set time to do this, Sofie suggests massaging your face for 30 seconds on each side. This motion isn't only stress-relieving: "The great thing is you're bringing blood and circulation into your skin, and that brings a luminescence," she says. If you're having an extra-sluggish day or had a super-salty meal, you can massage from the neck up to flush out the lymph nodes. "You can really open up the channels for bloat to drain—it's super effective."

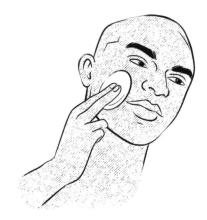

3. TOOL TIME.

Those who want to graduate to expert level can invest in beauty tools like *gua sha* or a jade roller, but you could even use a shot glass or, of course, your own two fingers (Sofie suggests curling your ring and middle fingers into the shape of a claw to mimic the shape of a roller tool). Use any of these tools while following the motions outlined above!

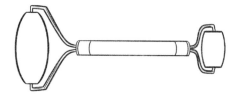

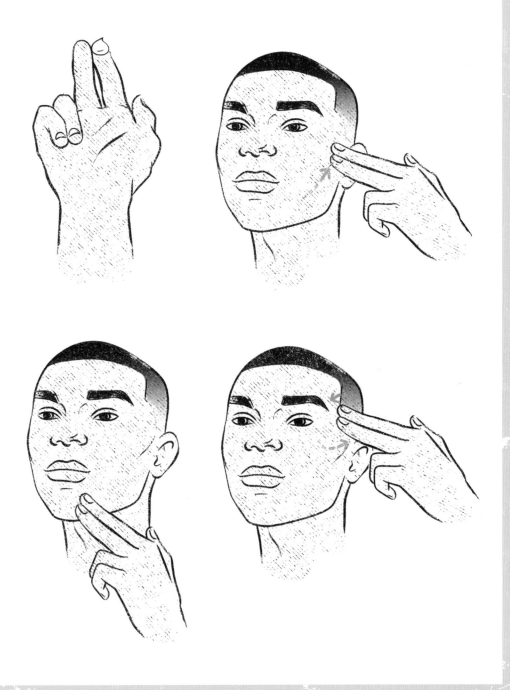

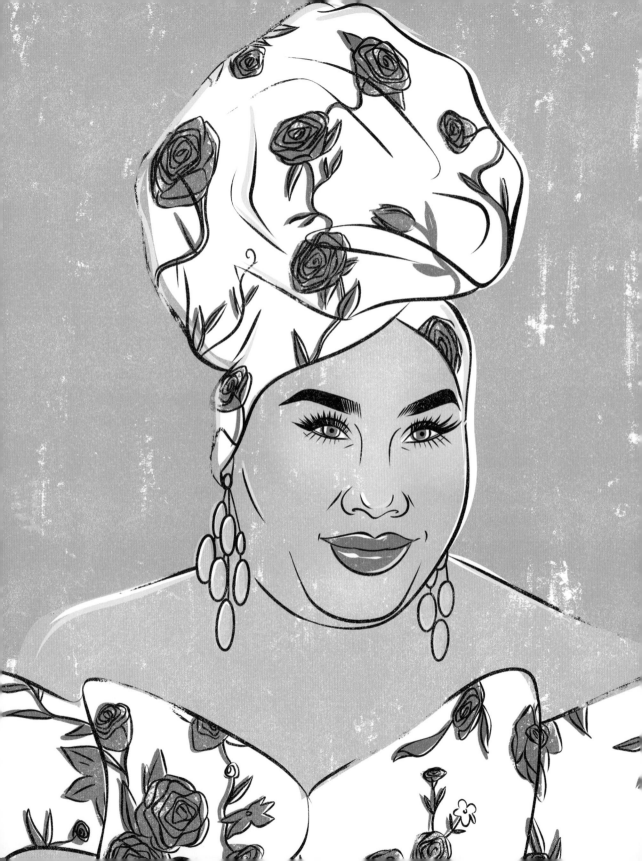

PATRICK STARRR

(1 9 8 9 -)

*From behind the MAC counter to
the front of its campaign.*

(A S   T O L D   T O   T H E   A U T H O R .)

MY PARENTS IMMIGRATED FROM THE PHILIPPINES TO NEW YORK City . . . then left for Florida for more space for their children. We were really lucky to have grown up there. There was lots of time to wander and dream. My favorite memories are of playing Chopin or Beethoven, translating how loud or soft I could interpret them. But as it turns out, the piano wasn't the only place I used my hands.

I bonded with my mom, Mama Starrr, with those same hands. I loved putting my fingers through her hair, pampering her after work. She was a traveling nurse and worked around the clock with her patients, many of them amputees. I understood firsthand about sacrifice from her. Knowing she had hard days, I wanted her to feel her best when she came home. I'd cut her nails, paint them, I'd comb her hair until it shined. She didn't have a plethora of beauty products back then, so she really didn't do much makeup. It was her base, a little bit of lipstick, blush, and bronzer. To me, my mom was beautiful.

Of course, my dad knew what we were up to. He wasn't thrilled that his oldest boy was beautifying his mother. Boys weren't supposed to play with makeup. They weren't supposed to play with their mother's hair. I remember my mom would succumb to my dad's opposition.

Back then, I thought they were being judgmental, but looking back now, I know they were protecting me from the world. They never hated me. Rather, they feared societal intolerance and the pain it could bring me.

And so I continued doing beauty on the side in secret. To make my own money, I started working, teaching piano lessons with a couple of clients. But the real money came from high school where I operated an underground beauty studio of sorts. I was a one-stop shop, all learned from blogs. Friends requested photoshoots for their quinceañeras, prom, headshots for drama club, or senior pictures. I was doing homecoming hair behind my parents' backs and would have a backpack of hot rollers I'd take to school. There, I'd give girls updos, high ponytails, put pins in them, take their photos, and send them away for prom. This was pre-YouTube and there weren't any tutorials, so I was self-taught and had to imagine what looked best. Soon, I was so in demand and started charging $25 for a photoshoot. I'd edit pictures in my parents' minivan almost like a shady deal, burn CDs in the park with the photos, and shell it out.

All along, I knew what I was lacking. As much as I'd become known as the go-to beauty guru at school, I knew to become successful I needed to get out of my shell. I was gay, shy, didn't socialize much . . . I needed to interact with people, engage with them, and boss up. So I did by getting a job at Panera, as a cashier. It was working there that I started developing this inner confidence. If I think about all of my jobs then, from being a full-time student, a piano teacher, Panera worker, hairstylist, makeup artist, photographer—it would all foreshadow what I'd do later. I just didn't know that I'd get there so soon.

I finally gained the courage to learn more about beauty and take it seriously. Only problem was, there wasn't a makeup academy near me. The next best thing, I figured, was finding a job behind a makeup counter. I applied to Ulta and Sephora, never heard back. I applied to MAC, the most intimidating one of them all, and yep, never heard back. It didn't surprise me. MAC was so glamorous, a store where they all wore black, were always so put together and beautiful—intimidating for a little chubby Filipino boy like me. It took all the courage for me, wearing my American Eagle cargo shorts and Abercrombie shirt, to even walk in and apply.

Months later, I was walking around and saw that MAC had an event for its Wonder Woman collection. I so happened to have my portfolio with me of my own photography, my own makeup, and had to seize the moment and show it to a manager. She looked over my book, wrote down my number, and said she'd be in contact.

I started working at the Macy's MAC at the mall, which was so different from an actual MAC store. But I was freaking out—I had made it! Of course, I was only freelance—only part-time—but I was on call and grateful to be there. I quickly learned how to sell, be enterprising, and learn the ropes of retail. For instance, to sell-through products, we had "theme days." So on Saturdays to sell out makeup, you'd dress up.

The theme for that day was time period makeup. I remember they asked me to do this crazy rock-and-roll boy-glam makeup. In my mind, this was redemption. I could wear makeup in public and be loud, be proud and celebrated. Unfortunately, when a manager saw me, she asked me to take it all off. "It's inappropriate," she said, referring to the fact that I was a man.

It hurt. This was a brand that I thought would accept me regardless of who I was. After all, their mantra was all sexes all ages all races. I felt shame, too. But I didn't have time to think about it so much. I knew if I brought it up I'd have my hours taken away from me. At that moment I was like, alright be calm. You gotta play the game to *make* the game.

So I played. I was able to play it so well that I garnered lots of sales, built a lot of relationships, and kept focused. To me, MAC was like going to Hogwarts, and I looked around to find the witches and wizards who could teach me. This one girl was really good at concealer, that other person was great at eyebrows, and that guy over there was really good at color theory. I would watch their makeup wizardry quietly, taking mental notes.

Meanwhile, something called YouTube was really kicking off. I remember putting a few videos up and not thinking so much about it. My Instagram started to grow as well, from 0 to 30,000, which was huge. I'd upload photos of my makeup looks wearing foundation, bronzer, blush, a little mascara. It was all very natural. At the time I was also making a lot of friends in the beauty industry. I decided to fly out to Los Angeles to a convention called the PHAME Expo. My friend Jenny69 picked me up from the airport and my former coworker at MAC, Steven, came to meet us. It was such an amazing experience to go from Florida to glamorous LA. At the expo, I met so many different creatives and moguls. It was the first time I was like, wow, I think I can make this influencer thing work.

In 2014 I took my YouTube channel really seriously, posting consistently. By then, my followers had grown to over 200,000. In between I was going back and forth to Los Angeles. Suddenly, my YouTube exploded, and in 2015, I was a finalist for an award called the NYX Face Awards. It was a competition where influencers could apply online, do makeup challenges, and the top six would compete for a $25,000 cash prize. But everyone else who didn't win would still get $10,000. In my head I was like, okay, I only need to win the $10,000 to help me fund a living in LA. Somehow, I manifested it and I walked away with what I set out to get. But I knew I needed a sign to tell me I was on the right path.

After the competition, I walked on a bridge on Hollywood and Highland where you could see the Hollywood sign. It was a gorgeous day, one where I felt that I wanted to move there. When I looked at my emails I realized I'd just gotten something from Sephora. When I opened it I screamed. It was the sign I was looking for. Sephora wanted me to be the new face of their nail campaign.

I moved to LA and everything became a blur. I was at Sephora, then landed an NYX holiday campaign, and eventually reached over 1 million followers. In 2016 I became the most-viewed beauty influencer, according to Google, and my videos were in the top five most watched next to Taylor Swift, Selena Gomez, Justin Bieber, and Bretman Rock. I was like, *this is so stupid*. Why am I, this little Filipino boy all the way from Astoria, Queens, and Orlando, being celebrated as one of the most viewed beauty influencers of 2016?

But everything came full circle later when my past came to my present. It was MAC Cosmetics that then approached me to be the face of their beauty campaign. I got goose bumps, I got chills. When I walked onto the set for the campaign, there was Mariah Carey casually gliding past us. I soon realized the campaign would be with her. Mariah. Carey. I couldn't believe what was happening, and it all was so disorienting. Was this real life?

I looked back at where I started from, that same chubby kid wearing cargo shorts, begging for a job at MAC. A flashback came where I remembered some people telling me I had to wipe off my makeup and hide who I was to work behind the counter. All of that shame, all of that sadness. But it was all worth it. The universal unfolded and I was back to where I started. This time, in front of the counter for all millions of people to see. Me, my makeup, and who I always was.

HOW TO BECOME A STARRR

Want to become a beauty guru? Here are Patrick Starrr's top tips to becoming your own, well, star.

1. WHO ARE YOU?
To become your own mogul, you have to know who you are first. At least, according to Patrick, who says, "Being self-aware is the very first step. It's understanding who you are and what you want to become." It's also knowing how to turn it into a business. "What's your purpose and objective?"

2. BUILD YOURSELF.
Take the time to build your makeup skills and communication abilities. "Become an expert and build experience. Own it," says Patrick.

3. CONSISTENCY PAYS OFF.
Patrick went from 0 to 30,000 followers on Instagram by posting regularly. He also took his YouTube seriously. "Don't lose focus on the goal and being consistent, amplifying your voice and doing everything from the groundwork will pay off."

4. COLLABORATE.
The biggest beauty gurus know that to shine, they need to work together. Which is why there are so many cameos when it comes to creating videos. Beauty influencers need each other. Don't be afraid to network, Patrick says. "Reach out to people who love the same thing as you do and keep them close."

5. BE Y-O-U.
Want to have longevity? Love what you do—and it'll show. From there, you can expand your empire. "For me, I expanded to television, different shows like on Snapchat, to even making music," Patrick says. "It's all interconnected—it's beauty after all. And it's genuinely what I'm passionate about."

"This time, in front of the counter for all millions of people to see.

ME, MY MAKEUP, and WHO I ALWAYS WAS."

— PATRICK STARRR

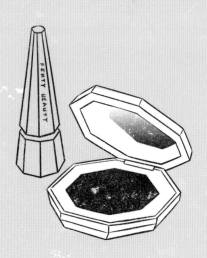

BAD BUNNY

(1 9 9 4 -)

Machismo is getting nailed.

THE INTERNET WAS SHAKEN WHEN THE PUERTO RICAN RAPPER Bad Bunny released the video for "Yo Perreo Sola." The song, the title of which translates to "I Twerk Alone," became an instant viral hit for its overwhelming dedication to female empowerment. "Te llama si te necesita / Ella perrea sola," Bad Bunny raps. ("She'll call you if she needs you / She twerks alone.") As he explained to *Rolling Stone,* "I wrote it from the perspective of a woman. I wanted a woman's voice to sing it—'yo perreo sola'—because it doesn't mean the same thing when a man sings it. But I do feel like that woman sometimes." Not only was it unusual for a rapper to be vocal about women's rights, but his latter statement perked up a few million ears. Was Bad Bunny, one of the hottest young rappers in the world, admitting that his gender wasn't so clearly defined?

The campy music video for the single seems to answer this question. Bad Bunny is in full drag—big boobs, cinched waist, enviable butt. Sporting multiple outfits, the star embodies femininity with ease, licking his lips, swaying his hips, and strutting in red patent leather heels and matching lipstick almost as if he does this every night. From long, wavy locks to a blond wig and beret, Bad Bunny's gender-bending itself might be nothing new—this book has *countless* examples from throughout history—but for a Latin trap and reggaeton artist to present himself as hyperfeminine isn't only fearless, it's revolutionary (though some in the LGBTQIA community have since questioned his motives accusing him of "queerbaiting," that is, appropriating gay lifestyle and pop culture to gain attention). In a culture bound to

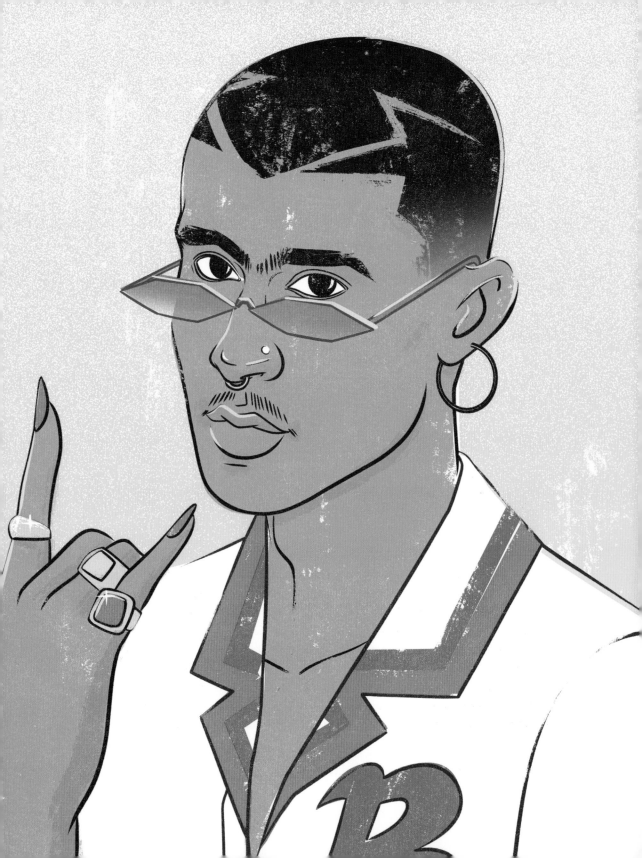

strict Catholicism, Latin patriarchy, and hypermasculine tradition, Bad Bunny is chipping away at toxic structures with signature sharp acrylic claws and sharper lyrics. This Puerto Rican star is fighting against misogyny, sexual violence, and homophobia, and becoming a defiant agent of change.

....

ON A TALK SHOW NOT TOO LONG AGO, BAD BUNNY MADE HEAD-lines for wearing a black kilt, but it was his shirt that got people talking. "They killed Alexa, not a man with a skirt," the T-shirt said, referencing the murder of Alexa Negrón Luciano, a homeless transgender woman. The country has been rife with several high-profile murders of members from LGBTQIA communities, and Luciano's brutal killing left many raw, including Bad Bunny, who once left a world tour to march alongside advocates against injustices. Traditional Latinx hip-hop has been, at times, particularly violent towards not only women but the LGBTQIA community as well—in 2019, an openly gay rapper named Kevin Fret was murdered in San Juan. Of course, open displays of hatred toward marginalized communities isn't unique to Puerto Rico. The pressures of being male in any hypermasculine culture is suffocating.

So it's all the more extraordinary that Bad Bunny is challenging Latinx machismo by championing those who live outside its realm of acceptability, and by expanding his own expression of gender and masculinity in spite of the potential physical or professional danger of doing so.

The rapper made headlines in 2018 when, after an award show in Miami, he'd passed by manicurists at a salon and decided he wanted to paint his nails, too. The next day, with a fresh coat of scintillating paint, he uploaded a photo of his fingers to Instagram. The photo went viral, with some detractors accusing him of "sexual deviance," in addition to applause.

Nails became his signature. He's shown painting his nails black in the video for "Estamos Bien." In the video for "Caro," Bad Bunny gets his nails done while wearing a bathrobe, then proceeds to blow on them, waiting for them to dry. He used Instagram to flaunt his oil-spilled talons for his millions of followers. He put a Spanish nail salon on blast on Twitter for refusing to paint his nails because he was a man. On the cover of PAPER magazine in 2019, his nails are long, almond-shaped, acrylic, and fierce as hell. But with great nails comes responsibility. His aesthetic had a political meaning as well—for instance, in "Caro," he casts people from all backgrounds: cis straight women, trans women, drag queens, a woman with Down syndrome. The same video shows a man kissing Bad Bunny's cheek. Homophobic statements would be roundly denounced. "Homophobia in this day and age, how embarrassing, loco," Bad Bunny would say after a rapper made homophobic statements about him.

While Bad Bunny has a larger-than-life persona and look, his words are grounded, level-headed, and impactful—and what can be more macho than such utter security in one's own authenticity, and a wholehearted belief in beauty and freedom of expression for all?

HOW TO PAINT YOUR CLAWS

At-home manicures are now just three strokes away.

Like Bad Bunny, you can perfect the art of painting your nails in the comfort of your own home. We enlisted the help of South Korea's biggest nail artist, Park Eunkyung, better known as Unistella to the hundreds of thousands of fans who follow her on social media. When she isn't creating the chicest creations for her clients—who include BLACKPINK, Sunmi, and TWICE, among many other celebrities—she's wowing international audiences with her unique, over-the-top creations. With her "glass nails," nail ice, wired nails, nail lights, even delectable Oreo nails, Park is inspiring a new generation of enthusiasts to get some fierce claws. But don't worry if you're not ready for anything *too* wild—on the following pages, Park maps out the foundations of nail-painting.

1. NAIL CHECK.

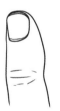

Before Park paints anything, she'll examine a client's nails. "We pay attention to the health of the nails as much as possible," she says. What does that even mean? Chances are, you already know: They're clear and shiny, have luster, and are moisturized. Unhealthy nails can be too thin or thick, have ridges or bumps, or be yellow or sometimes even brown. Above is an example of what a healthy nail looks like: the distal edge, nail plate, lunula, and cuticle should all more or less show on your nail.

2. CLEAN YOUR TALONS.

Wash your hands and use a nail polish remover to create a clean canvas on your nails. "It's important that you wipe away any dirt or leftover polish," says Park. A nontoxic nail polish remover will do the trick.

3. FILE THIS FOR LATER.

If you haven't done so already, take a nail clipper and trim your nails to the length you want. Then take a file and buff away any rough edges.

4. CUTICLE CUTIE.

Use a cuticle remover and cuticle stick to remove any dead skin cells. Gently remove skin to show off your beautiful lunulas, the white half-moon at the base of your nails.

5. ONE, TWO, THREE-STROKE.

If you're new to painting your nails, Park says to try using just three strokes to cover each nail. "You want the polish to really do the work, so don't feel you have to paint all over," she says. Instead, first paint down the center of the nail, then paint to the left of that first stroke, and finally to the right. "Press the brush from the base of the nail out to the top, don't be afraid to really go for it."

6. ACE THE BASE.

When you're ready to paint, put on a clear base coat first. "Think of a base like a primer," Park says. "It'll allow your polish to stay on longer." Take your brush and apply the base coat using the three-stroke method you've now "mastered,"—or something close to what makes you feel joy—then let it dry before applying color.

7. CUE THE Q-TIP.

Use the three-stroke method to apply color to each nail. Let this coat dry before moving on to the next step. Whether you're using just one color or a different one for each fingernail, don't be afraid to express yourself! Or to paint outside the lines. If that happens, simply take a little polish remover and clean up the edges. A good hack is to take a Q-tip and dip it in nail polish remover, then gently use it as an eraser.

8. NAILED IT.

Some nail professionals will say you can skip this step, but then again, if you already used a base, why not go for a top coat, too? Park says this will ensure that there's less chipping, as well as keep your nails shining longer. Clean up any wobbly mistakes and let your nails dry. After a few minutes, your claws will be ready to play!

YOU'VE GOT NAIL

*History's obsession with nails,
from fingers to toes.*

3200 BCE

Ur So Fierce

It's potentially your last day on Earth: How do you spend it? If you were an ancient Babylonian military man, you would be primping and pampering yourself at a salon.

A 1950s report of a royal excavation in Ur, the southern part of Babylonia, found that high-ranking army officials all carried a solid gold box with them. Estimated to be from 3200 BCE, the box was a manicure set, which included a spoon, pick, and tweezers. Before going into battle, these military personnel hit the salon to get ready and "could easily spend several hours having [their] hair lacquered and curled." They'd then have their nail polish applied, color-coordinated with their lips and eyes, by beauticians. In fact, pampering was a requirement. "No man of importance would permit himself to be seen in public unless he had been beautified," the same report described.

By the time these men arrived on the battlefield, their faces were snatched, their hair flawless, and their nails painted, showing their enemies that they didn't come to play. They came to *work*.

As far as memory extends, humans have always been fascinated with the opaque hardened shells—made of keratin, the same protein that forms the cells of our hair—that protect our fingertips while they're hard at work. Here are some unique and nail-biting stories of people through the centuries who nailed it when it came to their nails.

3000 BCE   ~400 BCE

The Emperor's New Glue

According to some accounts, before we had gels, acrylics, and French tips, Chinese emperors were the first to adopt the use of false nails. These were made from a robust mix of beeswax, egg white, gelatin, and rubber formed into an enamel. Only the elite were allowed to grow out their nails, as a sign of their royal class. With beautiful fingers like *these,* one couldn't possibly be bothered with manual labor.

Henna Henny

Henna has been used as a coloring agent for centuries, especially for decorating the palms, hands, feet, and nails. While it's associated with women in Middle Eastern, South Asian, and North and West African cultures, men have been known to wear henna as well. Henna mixed with indigo could be used to make a deep black dye for hair, but many men used the dye to decorate their nails. The nail dye was created by drying fresh henna leaves, sometimes with indigo, and grinding them into a powder, then mixing the powdered henna with water and lemon and lime juices to create a paste. The paste would be applied to the fingers and left for 6 to 12 hours, covered with a damp cloth or a leaf. The result: a semipermanent stain that would dazzle for weeks on end.

> *The Roman historian Pliny the Elder once studied nails, concluding they were "the termination of sinews," aka dried-up muscles that protruded through fingers and toes.*

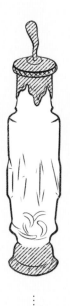

File This for Later

In Norse mythology, the end times, or Ragnarok, was prophesied as culminating in an epic battle between the gods and the spirits of dead warriors, with life ending when a ship full of dead people—and disembodied fingernails—appear to take you into the next lifetime. Needless to say, these Nordic folks kept their nails very short.

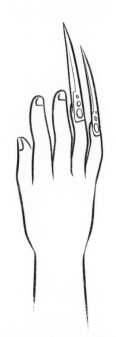

800s CE ········· 1200s CE ········ 1348–1644 ·········

Holy Nails

In the Middle Ages, it was essential for kings, popes, noblemen, and anyone in a position of power to have reliquaries in their possession. Reliquaries were the physical remains of saints, everything from bones to clothing to body hair and or nail clippings. It all started in 809, when the Abbot of the Monastery of Elnon, founded by Saint Amandus, patron saint of Belgium, cut a deceased saint's nails, in the hopes that they'd look their best when arriving in the kingdom of heaven. While he may have had good intentions, it inspired a creepy capitalistic business. Gravediggers began cutting the beards, teeth, and toenails of other purported saints and selling them as sacred relics. The most famous of these may be nail clippings from Saint Clare, found in a crystal flask dating from the fourteenth century.

Everything I Touch Is Literal Gold

Midas touch? More like the Ming bling. Like their ancestors more than four thousand years before them, the men of the Ming dynasty wouldn't buff or clip their nails, often growing them out, long and sharp. The royal family flaunted their talons in reds and blacks, and silver and gold dust would even be applied to their nails. Both royal men and women also wore trendy spiked nail guards that were as fashionable as they were threatening. These guards could be up to 6 inches long, were made of solid gold and accessorized with precious stones, and fit right on top of the wearer's finger, so that anything a royal touched was *literal* gold.

Cuticle Cutie

The gendering of nails and their maintenance stemmed from the Victorian era, during which a stark binary between men and women was created in Western culture. Women were required to be more domestic, remaining indoors to keep up their households. Northam Warren, who created the formula for Cutex Cuticle Remover, capitalized on fearmongering to grow his business, warning women that if they didn't care for their hands, they were "low-class." Cutex created maintenance products for cuticles and nails, and eventually launched a line of liquid nail tints, though these didn't catch on until the 1920s (at which time the company also introduced an acetone-based polish remover).

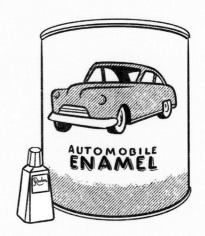

1830   1911   1920s

Hang In There

Manicures as a treatment can first be traced to the nineteenth century. In France, King Louis-Philippe hired a podiatrist named Monsieur Sitts to aid him with all his foot ailments. One of Monsieur Sitts's tasks was to remove the king's hangnails. At first, the entire process wasn't perceived as a beauty treatment, but rather one of necessity and health. But soon, it became a royal trend to have your hands and feet groomed—a precursor to the modern manicure.

Rev Your Engines

Before the early 1920s, nail polishes weren't "polishes" at all—instead, they were colored stains or powders. A French makeup artist named Michelle Menard would change all that. Menard worked for Charles Revson, his brother Joseph, and chemist Charles Lachman. Their business was called Revlon (a combination of the three cofounders' names). Taking inspiration from the durable, glossy paint used on cars, Menard created an enamel from the same nitrocellulose lacquer used to paint cars, but with a lot less strength. The result: a revolutionary nail polish that would change the course of history. Revlon began selling this new "nail polish" in 1932, and Hollywood helped propel it forward as a must-have beauty item for women.

Need an Extension

What do root canals and fingernail extensions have in common? Absolutely nothing. But for the sake of this section, we're going to say everything—if not for a certain dentist/inventor, we wouldn't have the dramatic looks that acrylic nails create. One day, Philadelphia dentist Dr. Slack painfully broke a nail. He used materials from his clinic to remedy the missing piece, patching it up with a piece of aluminum foil and dental acrylic. He awoke the next day to a surprise: not only was there no more pain, but the acrylic nail looked natural. After experimenting with acrylic monomers and polymers, he created the perfect product to not only strengthen nails but extend them as well. He patented his invention, and would go on to create other innovations in nail care, including UV-cured gels, fiberglass-reinforced polymers, light-activated liquids, and more.

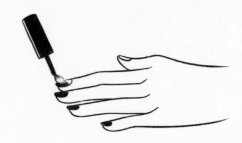

1950s ····· 2000s

Piece of Work

By the turn of the twentieth century, nails were becoming a means of accessible expression. "Man salons," the biggest trend of the early aughts, provided guys with *man*icures, promoting the idea that a hypermasculine space would make men comfortable with grooming. At the same time, nail salons grew into big business, with nail art driving profits. Today, nail innovations abound: stickers, holographic foils, crackle effects, multiple textures that come in beads, sandlike polishes, and more. And nontoxic, "all-natural" polishes have since debuted on the market, with several companies eliminating known carcinogens including formaldehyde, dibutyl phthalate, and toluene, so you can get cute cuticles without having to harm yourself or the world around you. The best part? Dressed-up nails and nail maintenance are no longer associated with one particular gender—some of today's swaggiest stars, from Harry Styles (see page 207) to Bad Bunny (see page 160) to Lil Nas X, and young folks around the world enjoy having color at their fingertips.

YOU'LL ALWAYS NAIL IT WHEN YOU EMBRACE YOURSELF FOR WHO YOU ARE.

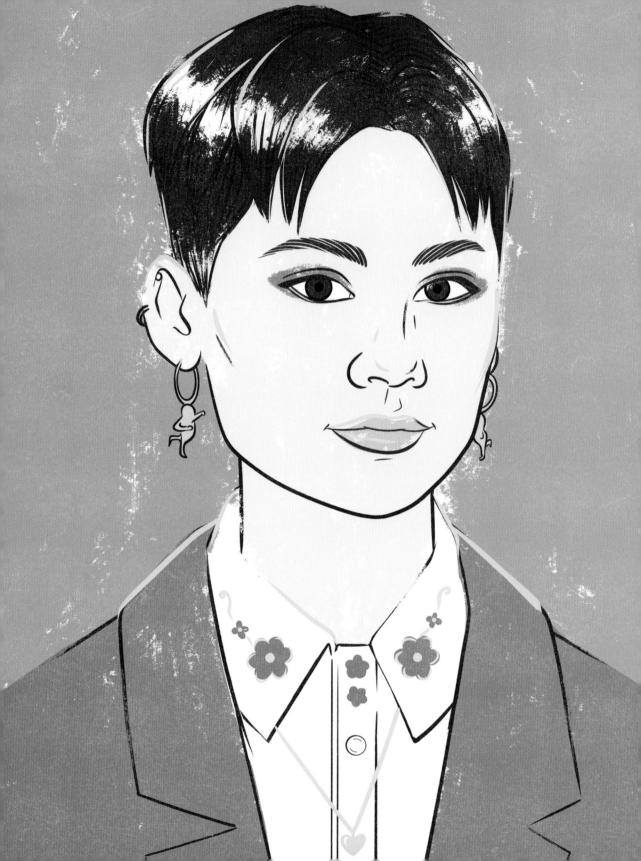

IAN ALEXANDER

(2 0 0 1 -)

*How beauty allowed him to finally
come out to the world.*

(A S   T O L D   T O   T H E   A U T H O R .)

I GREW UP IN A MILITARY FAMILY. MY DAD WORKS FOR THE government, so we moved around a lot. I grew up in Hawaii and Japan and the DC area so I experienced many cultures as an American foreigner. My mom is Vietnamese and my father is white, so I come from a biracial household. In Vietnamese culture, there is less emphasis on makeup for all genders, but beauty is still an essential part of Vietnamese culture. For men, beauty standards have changed a lot over the centuries and, at one point, long hair was a sign of beauty and wealth for men—which goes to show that the gender binary and beauty standards are literally just social constructs.

My parents are very religious, which means they're very heteronormative and cisnormative. Not all religious people are heteronormative, but for those familiar with the Mormon or Latter Day Saints faith, that religion is based off the values of cis, white, straight men. I was raised with this idea that male masculinity is tough: they're strong and they don't show emotion; female means that you're nurturing and you take care of the children. It didn't allow me a lot of room for expression except in my femininity, so I felt like I had a lot of room to explore dresses and makeup, stuff like that.

When I came out, I was thirteen. I had a really difficult time coming out to my parents, so I wrote a letter because I didn't know how to articulate my feelings. I slid it under their door and a few minutes later my dad came out. He was very upset, angry, confused. It was confusion and also concern as a parent, thinking that I'd be mistreated and discriminated against. My parents could not get past the idea of other people's perceptions of gender. They were afraid of me being excluded because I was different.

Makeup was socially acceptable while I was identifying as female for the first, like, twelve years or so of my life. Once I figured out that I actually felt more like a boy, I still enjoyed makeup and what were considered feminine things, which led to pushback from my parents. "I don't get it. You're not a boy because you like pink. You like makeup. You like all these girly things," they'd say. They had always known me as being obsessed with princesses and dressing up like one. I remember when I was like three or four putting on makeup with a little lip gloss palette. I would kind of do it on my eyes, lips, and cheeks. I was beating my face when I was a toddler.

Makeup has always been part of who I am. We know that makeup has no gender. Beauty is just another form of self-expression...

This love for beauty carried into the rest of my childhood. I very much enjoyed dressing up in frilly things. I then went through an emo phase. Around age twelve, I started dressing up in all black. Suddenly, my beauty went from pink and glittery to thick black eyeliner, black lipstick, and very pale foundation—dark goth. It was all about using makeup as a way to express my personality, and what I was feeling on the inside. I was very shy and socially anxious, and I didn't speak a lot—so most people saw my personality through how I look.

I got into makeup more seriously when I was fourteen. Interestingly, it's also when I was the most insecure about people's perceptions of me. I finally came out publicly as trans and I wasn't wearing makeup to school anymore. I felt insecure about people's perceptions and invalidations of my gender. All along, I still wanted to wear makeup, so I kind of did it in secret. I would spend hours doing a very extravagant makeup look, take pictures in it, then immediately wash it off. For two years, until I was sixteen, I would do this alone in the bathroom, putting on over-the-top looks from drag makeup, to wearing huge, false lashes, to shaving my eyebrows. I did the whole thing.

I was also still hiding this from my parents. They had been so adamant when I came out to them that there was no way I could be a boy. This was the longest journey of self-acceptance for me: accepting that femininity was just as much a part of me as masculinity. I tried to tell them, "I'm just really flamboyant!"

"What will people think of you?" my parents would ask. "They're going to be mean to you at school." My father said a lot of really hurtful transphobic things. This inability to accept me for who I was triggered a long, deep depression. I felt lost and so unloved in my own home. It caused a lot of mental health problems. The only time I could be myself was when I went to school. There, people at least respected my gender identity and would say my name.

Meanwhile, I felt less alone thanks to the Internet and Tumblr. I came to research everything about my nonbinary masculine identity. I've since concluded that there's gender identity, which is internal, and gender expression, which is external, and how both of those can coexist. Someone can identify as a man and be wearing a long wig and full makeup with a dress.

This was all affirmed when I got the role of Buck Vu, a Vietnamese American trans high school student. The casting call on Tumblr and Twitter was for a fourteen- or fifteen-year-old Asian American trans actor. It was so specific and I checked off all of the boxes of what they were looking for. Sure enough, I got the role.

Being on *The OA* played such a transformative role in my life. It provided me with this opportunity to leave an environment that I felt was toxic, and also a chance for me to be celebrated for who I was. On set, everyone knew me solely as Ian, the boy, and didn't know me as anything prior to that. I was just myself and it was so surreal just to be in an environment where I was fully and wholeheartedly accepted. I really needed that. It really saved me.

Today, I think I definitely have felt a lot of pressure for trying to be the best role model I can be for trans teens, but I have grown into myself and loved and accepted the parts of myself that I feel are flawed. I'm trying to learn how to have more grace with myself and be patient and realize that I am allowed to make mistakes. I'm allowed to grow and learn.

Makeup has always been part of who I am. We know that makeup has no gender. Beauty is just another form of self-expression; it's the art form of painting your face. I love using makeup as a way to emphasize certain parts of my outfit. Because I have been very shy and insecure in my life, I feel like putting on makeup almost gives me this armor that I need to be more confident. Most recently, I've grown into being more comfortable with myself without makeup as well. I don't have to rely on it for my confidence—rather, it's this extra fun additional bonus. That being said, femininity has always been my favorite costume. It always feels like a safe space for me to play dress-up. There's a childlike joy we all deserve to explore in dressing up in a skirt or putting on a fancy makeup.

Pretty Ic

BOY BEAUTY TODAY
IS INHERENTLY
REBELLIOUS.

noclastic

THINK OF MEN WHO'VE KICKED MASCULINITY TO the curb, refused to play by the gender binary, and lived and looked as authentically as they could: the likes of David Bowie, who came out as bisexual at a time when it wasn't embraced; Prince, who was villainized for being outwardly sexual; and BTS, who've been criticized by Western audiences for daring to wear makeup; among many others. While rulers and aristocrats may have been the rock stars of their times, we start to see beauty heroes come in the form of artists, pop culture figures, and everyday people, especially in the present. Here's to the rule-breakers, the antiestablishment iconoclasts who weaponized beauty for positive change, leading the charge in the identity revolution.

LORD BYRON

(1 7 8 8 - 1 8 2 4)

This sex symbol faced his self-esteem publicly.

IT'S SAID THAT MAN CANNOT LIVE ON BREAD ALONE. BUT that's exactly how nineteenth-century England's hottest celebrity, Lord Byron, sustained himself. With pursed lips, curly Grecian hair, and a lean body, the best-selling author had millions of admirers who fawned over his every move. He was so broodingly handsome both men and women were advised to stay away. "Bad, mad and dangerous to know," wrote a certain Lady Caroline Lamb in a diary entry from 1812. "But that beautiful pale face is my fate . . ."

A lothario who broke hearts with abandon, George Gordon Noel, aka Lord Byron, was a prolific writer known for seducing anyone he wanted to. Yet behind his veneer of confidence was a man who struggled with body image and low self-esteem—so much so that he'd attempt to alter his aesthetics in the extreme, putting himself on a strict diet of thin bread and tea.

Born with a clubfoot, he was bullied as a child and made into a pariah, an experience he'd write about later. When he came into adulthood, he traveled the world, soaking in experiences in exotic locations like Greece and Albania and taking in the foreign cultures, which would inspire his many books of fiction and poetry.

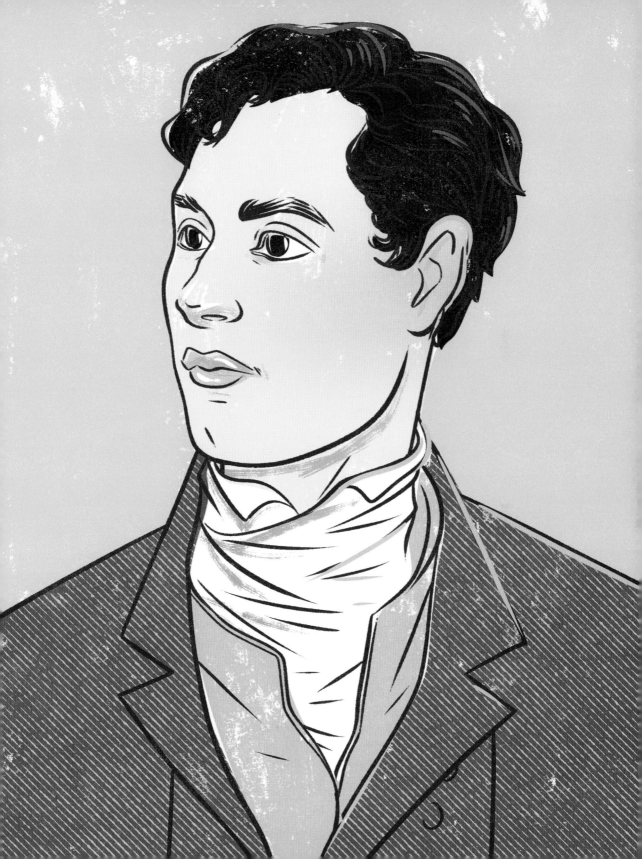

But when he came back to London, the teasing did not cease. He was still demeaned as the man who went about town wearing an orthopedic shoe. He turned to sex as a means to cope with his self-esteem—he was known to carry dozens of condoms wherever he went, and didn't discriminate by gender. His sexual proclivities were only enhanced by his rise to stardom after the publication of his poetry, including longer works like *Don Juan* and *Childe Harold's Pilgrimage.* He was thrust into the national spotlight and became a certified celebrity. And with so much attention, the pressure he felt to look a certain way increased.

He was obsessed with his "morbid propensity to fatten," according to the book *Calories & Corsets,* and when he'd look in the mirror, he was disgusted by his figure. Such self-hatred led to dangerous eating habits and an extreme workout regimen. When he wasn't eating, he was thinking of ways to lose weight, often layering himself in heavy woolen clothing and exercising so he'd sweat his weight off.

By his mid-twenties, Lord Byron was suffering from severe dysmorphia, going so far as to destroy any painting of himself that wasn't up to his standards. He lived every day obsessing over every inch of his image. Many accounts recall him even secretly curling his hair every night to achieve that wavy-haired, Grecian appearance. According to one story, Lord Byron's friend Scrope Berdmore Davies caught him one night with curl-papers. "But you have succeeded admirably in deceiving your friends, for it was our conviction that your hair curled naturally," he allegedly said to Byron. "Yes, naturally every night," replied Byron. "But do not let the cat out of the bag, for I am as vain of my curls as a girl of sixteen."

Unfortunately, rumors of his beautifying habits, along with his sexual preferences, soon permeated British society. The media hounded him for being distastefully superficial and questioned him about his sexuality. Newspapers began circulating stories of his affairs with his half-sister, and articles on whether he was homosexual (illegal at the time, and punishable by death). At this point, Lord Byron decided it would be easier to leave it all behind.

On the morning of April 25, 1816, he fled the country and was painted by newspapers as being forced out in exile. After leaving England, he adopted Greece as his home, and traded in his career as a writer for one as a revolutionary. Becoming a Greek citizen, he fought for the country's independence from the Ottoman Empire during the Greek War of Independence. But tragedy would strike on the battlefield—he would die from a fever at the age of thirty-six.

Years later, we remember Lord Byron for his brilliant written works, his genius poetry and prose, which are still revered as literary treasures. However, his struggles with his self-esteem and experiences with body dysmorphia are buried, as if they make his legacy any less important. Disordered eating, anxiety, and low self-esteem are part of the masculine and non-female experience, today propelled by each celebrity-endorsed diet and Instagram "fit tea" ad, and the homogeneity of representation in media. Lord Byron was forced to repress his feelings of shame and self-hatred—there was little language and dialogue for what he was struggling with during his time. These days, negative body image is an ongoing conversation, but it's heartening to know there are champions of change, body-positivity advocates, and more and more people speaking out about their experiences with dysmorphia. If Lord Byron lived today, he would certainly be able to find others who celebrated him for the entirety of his being, and people who could help guide him toward accepting himself more fully.

If Lord Byron lived today, he would certainly be able to find others who celebrated him for the entirety of his being, and people who could help guide him toward accepting himself more fully.

BODY POSITIVITY

ABearNamedTroy on learning to love his body and how you can, too.

When it comes to the modern body positivity movement, women have led the demand for the expansion of beauty standards from the harmful and claustrophobic one-size-fits-all definitions. But when it comes to those of other genders, there's still a long way to go.

A recent study by the National Center for Biotechnology Information found that men experience body dysmorphia as much as women do. In a society that deems male bodies appealing only if they're lean, slim, or chiseled (though, there has been a movement to also spotlight dad bods), Troy Solomon is advocating for change, for space to promote healthier discussions around self-love and self-image.

His Instagram, @ABearNamedTroy*, has inspired thousands of men around the world to embrace their own unique bodies, to not shy away from their shapes, and to take pride in who they are. In the paragraphs that follow, he talks about how he came to gain confidence and acceptance, and how you can, too.

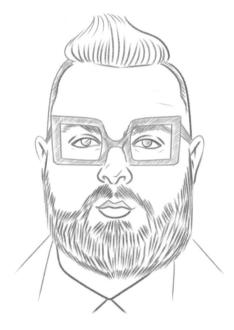

....

I definitely had a rough childhood when it comes to my body image. I was always on diets and my dad was definitely guilty of body-shaming me—but I also know that's very much a generational thing. Our parents weren't having the kinds of conversations we are having now in regard to self-acceptance and body positivity. But there were definitely cruel times in my life where the adults made me feel like my worth correlated with a number on a scale (and the higher it was, the less I was worth).

My stepmom was probably the worst and ultimate culprit when it comes to my experience with self-hate, body-shaming, and disordered eating. She was very strict on what times I could eat (she restricted me to not being able to eat past six p.m. because of a study Oprah shared that was geared toward women over the age of thirty—I was thirteen). She would hide food from me. She would give my stepsiblings different food than me. She was always constantly hyperfocused on my weight. I'm just glad I've been able to free myself from the damage of that trauma.

My journey to self-acceptance started with me coming out of the closet and accepting that part of me. It felt like all my secrets were gone. So from there I was giving myself the freedom to explore the rest of what I have to offer, which eventually led to body acceptance, and that acceptance grew into love. People think you just wake up one day and love yourself, but it's such a longer process than wishing upon a star.

As of this printing, @ABearNamedTroy has been rebranded to @lordtroy.

Everything changed when I came out in 2012, and my own exploration within the queer space as a bigger person, which, in the gay community is considered a "bear," allowed me to connect with my community. When I first really launched ABearNamedTroy, I never knew what it would amount to or what levels of self-acceptance it would take me to. I sort of just fell into the process of exposing myself for the world's consumption. I've always wanted to connect with people on a real level, and I think once I started noticing how I was able to connect with people just by being myself and sharing my self-exploration, I definitely felt this sense of responsibility to be open and honest with my audience. We have a really special bond, and they've seen more of my body (and soul) than a lot of people I know in real life—and I'm super excited to continue sharing new parts of me with them and continuing to grow that connection.

The relationship I have with my body is the longest one I've ever been in. I'd be lying if I said every day was easy, but I do think I've reached a point where I can have that conversation with myself when I'm feeling low and get down to the root of why I'm really feeling that way. And, without fail, every single time, it never has to do with my body. I think being super self-aware and self-analytical has gotten me to this point of truly knowing none of my emotional issues have anything to actually do with how I look physically, and I try really hard to use that knowledge to continue my self-growth and exploration. It took many, many years of work—both unlearning through growth, and growing through unlearning.

Beauty, to me, is universal.

Everyone is physically beautiful. Because of how I genuinely feel, I really don't spend too much time thinking about physical beauty. I focus my attention on how beautiful you are on the inside and I think makeup allows us to express those parts of us in a visible way. Personally, I use beauty products as tools for creative expression. I feel like I mostly use makeup, combined with fashion, to tell a story. I think once you reach a true level of self-acceptance and self-love, your relationship with makeup changes for the better. It becomes less about hiding and more about freedom and empowerment.

If I were to give advice to someone it's this:

First start with acknowledging that you currently don't wholly accept yourself, and get to a comfortable place of accepting that. So many of us get fixated on the parts we don't like about ourselves and are so focused on fixing them that we don't take the time to accept that we don't like those parts of ourselves. Once you're there, and ready to work on it, spend intimate time with the part of yourself you have an issue with. That could mean staring in the mirror naked or journaling or meditating.

Therapy is also a great tool for learning how to fully embrace yourself. The only way to maintain power over your insecurity is by embracing it as part of you—start saying this mantra in the mirror:

"I accept you, you are a part of me, and I have the power."

From there, you'll start to understand where you're heading in your personal journey and that the process is different for everyone.

The LUGUBRIOUS TALES of BODY MODIFICATIONS PAST

Stories of plastic surgery to keep you up at night.

THERE WILL BE BLOOD . . . AND NIPS, TUCKS, STITCHES, AND cuts, too. While plastic surgery and other body and cosmetic enhancements are common-place in our modern world, when the field was in its nascent stages . . . let's just say it was absolutely gruesome. Thankfully, today, plastic surgery and body enhancements have come a long way in terms of both technology and stigmas. While these surgeries may have been created out of necessity—i.e., to reconstruct a face damaged in battle—patients today are frequently electing to undergo surgeries to feel more confident and better in their own skin. And in places like South Korea and Colombia, enhancements are commonplace. While plastic surgery may not be for everyone, if it helps you become more confident and happier, it shouldn't come with a stigma attached. On the following pages, we recount some of the wildest moments in the history of plastic surgery.

WARNING: THIS MAY GET A LITTLE TOO *REAL* FOR SOME.

600 BCE

A Nose for a Nose

Cheat on your spouse? Steal from your neighbor? If you lived in medieval India, punishment for such transgressions could mean losing your nose! The *Sushruta Samhita,* an ancient medical journal written in Sanskrit, describes a procedure that is now considered one of the earliest instances of plastic surgery. The method wasn't pretty, and involved using a flap of skin from a patient's forehead to reconstruct their nose.

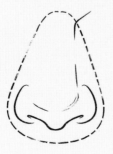

1415–1465

Armed and Ready

A Bavarian military surgeon named Heinrich von Pfalzpaint treated more than four thousand casualties during the siege of Marienberg Fortress. After seeing so many patients, the doctor developed a revolutionary method of nasal reconstruction. Though gruesome—not to mention seriously uncomfortable, as it involved grafting skin from the arm to the nose and keeping it there for eight to ten days—his method apparently worked. In fact, it was so effective, it was used on syphilis patients whose noses became deformed due to the progression of the disease, and continued to be used in these cases until the discovery of penicillin, the cure for syphilis, in 1928.

The Mad Scientist

Dr. Charles Conrad Miller first rose to prominence when he published one of the first modern-day articles detailing how to create an eye lift. He gained prominence and local fame as a cosmetic surgeon in the Chicago area, and treated many patients in those years.

But his methods were not medically sound—in fact, they were also downright dangerous. His sadistic practices included a painful, if not outright violent, procedure that corrected protruding ears by tying them flat to the head. He'd grind together rubber and gutta-percha (a plastic substance made from the latex of several species of Malaysian trees) and use the mixture as a facial filler. And when patients complained that their procedures didn't heal properly, the doctor would just scoff. As the years wore on, he developed "megalomaniacal and almost messianic egotism," and would treat patients "as if they were uniformly simple-minded." But in 1914, after a farmer died from ingesting pills he had gotten from a sham pharmacy run by Miller, the *Chicago Tribune* exposed the surgeon as a quack. He was charged with selling drugs without a prescription, but when the case came to trial, the plaintiff never arrived in court to testify, so Miller was free to go, an example of how unregulated the cosmetic surgery business was at the time.

1881–1950   1882–1960

Burn Notice

The first documentation of tragedy stemming from plastic surgery comes from the early 1900s. In an emergency procedure to save a burn victim, surgeon Harold Gillies attempted a skin transplant. The patient's body rejected the skin graft, leading to heart collapse and death. Gillies would go on to become the first man to perform successful skin grafts, however, and eventually even reconstructed a soldier's eyelids.

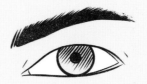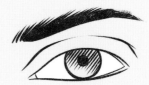

Seeing Double

Today, double eyelid surgery is common in most East Asian and Southeast Asian countries. The top destination for these procedures is South Korea, now the leading country when it comes to plastic surgery innovations. So popular is double eyelid surgery that in 2014, over 1.4 million people in South Korea alone underwent the procedure, which creates permanent creases or folds in monolids. While there are accusations that double eyelid surgery is popular because of East Asians' desire to look European, the actual story of double eyelids comes from Japan in 1886, when a Japanese ophthalmologist named Kotaro Mikamo, created the first procedure. Although accused of doing so as a "Westernizing" surgery, he later explained that wasn't true. "His intentions were to emulate the common unique Japanese aesthetic characterized by the double eyelid or *futae mubuta,* aka creating eyes that were common in Japanese people (yes, double eyelids *are* natural to East Asians and Southeast Asians as well, accounting for 50 percent of the population). In Korea this aesthetic is called *ssang-kk-upeul,* which literally means to "double cover," and it became popular thanks to the actress Hwang Shin-hye. With an oval face and bright, double-lidded eyes, she became a sensation in the 1980s. Today the procedure has become so commonplace in South Korea, young people request it after graduating from high school.

1886-PRESENT DAY ···· PRESENT DAY

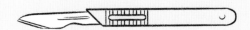

Butting into It

While facial procedures are popular in East Asia, body modifications have become commonplace in South America, namely in Colombia, the fourth-leading world destination for cosmetic surgeries. In 2018, more than 75,000 foreigners traveled to Bogotá for body enhancements, according to the International Society of Plastic Surgery. The most common procedures are breast implants, liposuction, and, more recently, butt implants. The latter increased in popularity by 252 percent from 2000 to 2015, and includes various procedures like a fat transfer, lift, and actual implants filled with hydrogel or silicone.

Going Under

In America, plastic surgery and body enhancements are becoming less stigmatized, largely because of the rise of social media. The American Society for Aesthetic Plastic Surgery reported that in 2015, 1.2 million men elected to go under the knife. That's triple the number from 1997. The most popular procedures were eye and neck lifts, as well as rhino-plasty (nose jobs), liposuction, and gynecomastia surgery (aka chest size reduction). While some may argue that it's empowering to receive surgery, others are more wary, arguing that natural bodies are beautiful as they naturally are. Whatever the case, do what's right for you—and only after extensive research. We've come a long way from the early days of plastic surgery, do keep in mind that while plastic surgery can help, it can still also harm.

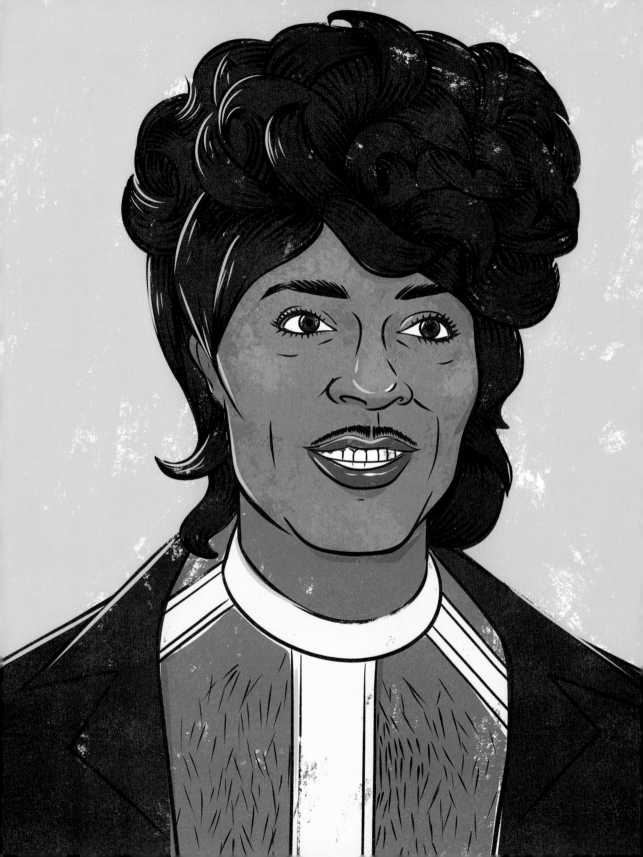

LITTLE RICHARD

(1 9 3 2 - 2 0 2 0)

The architect of rock and roll.

LEGENDARY ROCK STARS ALL HAD A SIGNATURE LOOK: PRINCE and his eyeliner, David Bowie with his Ziggy Stardust makeup, Elvis Presley and his synonymous coif. But these iconoclasts all had a singular inspiration in common: Little Richard. While history may have cemented these gods of music as iconoclasts, each took a note out of Little Richard's larger-than-life playbook. This self-proclaimed "architect of Rock and Roll" not only pushed a new genre of music forward, but was the very first modern artist to usher in a new era of colorful male self-expression. If higher hair brought you closer to God, Little Richard must have been mere inches away from Jesus's throne. He was doing God's work—and damn, he looked divine.

Prior to Little Richard's rise in the late 1950s, the Western world was black and white—literally, with men relegated to wearing only a bland set of monotone suits, shoes, ties, and shirts. The fifties were all about modest attire, and style meant that you looked squeaky clean, if not sterile. The typical man sported slicked-back hair, a clean-shaven face, looks free of any means of "deviant" expression. The biggest stars of the era personified this, and seemed near carbon copies of each other: white, cisgender, straight—like Buddy Holly and Chuck Berry, rockabilly artists who topped the charts in the fifties.

When Little Richard jumped onto the scene, he shocked the system, and would eventually make history as one of the only Black American men to dominate the Top 100, graciously painting the Billboard charts in a multitude of dazzling colors. He single-handedly revived pop culture and popular music. He awakened the world to a new era of masculinity—a beautiful, queer, southern Black man was about to change history.

But it wasn't all rainbows. Growing up Black, queer, and religious had many challenges, especially if you were born in the South, as Little Richard was. Singing gospel at churches and local functions, young Richard's voice began to stand out. His performances went so hard, his raw and rasping voice gravelly in microphone, that he eventually became noticed by a local gospel singer named Sister Rosetta Tharpe. She invited him to sing alongside her on stages, where Richard got his first taste of fame.

Around this time, Richard began expressing himself with beauty. "I used to call myself the Magnificent One," he said. "I was wearing makeup and eyelashes when no men were wearing that." He experimented with his hair, letting it hang, letting it grow, and braiding it in every which way. He'd take his mother's makeup, set it on his face, apply lipstick, and strut around town with his hips loosely swaying from side to side. He was living his authenticity and expressing his truth. This newfound freedom of expression didn't go over so well with his religious father, who later beat Richard for having the audacity to embrace his divine femininity. As Richard would later recall, his father abused him so badly, he fled his home. "He said he wanted seven boys, and that I had spoiled it because I was gay."

But the show always goes on. Richard worked traveling and minstrel shows for years, until he landed his first record deal at eighteen years old in 1951 and everything came together. That's when he met an equally vibrant queer performer who went by the name Esquerita, who became a pivotal figure in Little Richard's life and played a key role in the creation of his persona. Enamored by Esquerita's fierce energy and showstopping style, Richard would learn to play piano from him, perfect his growl and shout, and expand his musicality. Their femininity wasn't weakness; it was the superpower that allowed them to shine.

Onstage, Little Richard was free—he was fearless, enigmatic. He combined boogie-woogie with an essence of gospel and blues, while incorporating aesthetics from the period's traditional notions of masculine and feminine, and made the sum into a potpourri that was entirely his own. His unconventional style finally caught the eye of a music label and, unbeknownst to the world, would become the blueprint for rock and roll.

Little Richard's raw sound, full of hoots, hollers, and moans, was refreshingly sexual in an era that was all about buttoning up. And his persona, from his slicked-back coiffure and sparkling outfits to his fearlessness onstage shimmying, both entranced and shook the country. His biggest single would be 1955's "Tutti Frutti," a raucous love song that worried parents for its risqué lyrics. Richard's original lyrics were considered NC-17 back then: "If it's tight, it's alright. If it's greasy, it makes it easy." The song would be monumental as the first American hit alluding to gay sex.

In the years that followed, his persona grew even bigger. His hair got higher, his shoulder pads thicker, his razor-thin mustache but a line. He began expressing himself even more with his face, painting on Pancake 13 foundation (which would become his signature look) and smoldering his eyes with liners and shadows, while wearing outlandish wigs and exuberant outfits. Makeup on any man at the time had shock value, but Richard's usage wasn't just to make people stop and stare. It was, for a Black entertainer in predominantly white spaces, strategic as well. "I wore makeup and wild outfits to keep white people from focusing on me as some kind of a sexual threat," he told the *Wall Street Journal*. "I knew that if I looked crazy, not cool, I wouldn't be seen that way. And it worked. People focused on the music."

The next years would find Little Richard touring the world, no longer solely an American act, but an international one. He was so big, he even discovered new talent to open for him at his concerts, like a then little-known band called the Beatles. He later recalled teaching the group about rock and roll at a stop in Hamburg, Germany, even coaching Paul McCartney to sing his signature "Woo," in a high-pitched scream.

"Paul was so crazy about me," he recalled in a *Rolling Stone* interview. Others also took note, like Elvis Presley, who not only covered "Tutti Frutti" but also took aesthetic inspiration from Little Richard's hair and colorful suits. Prince would come next, his androgynous look and vocal style a nod to Little Richard's. And who could forget David Bowie, who said he thought he'd "heard God" in the rock-and-roller's voice, and gained courage from Richard to create his own iconic foundation-slathered persona.

While some of his protégés would become better known than others, Little Richard deserves a lot of credit. He was the *original,* in terms of music, and a trendsetter both aesthetically and, perhaps more important, culturally. He created outlandish, ostentatious looks with fearless sexuality and was often criticized for it. It was unfair, as his flair was later co-opted by white rockers and deemed not only "cool," but acceptable. While Elton John could wear a sparkly coat and Elvis could sway his hips, it had been considered unsightly for a Black man like Little Richard to do so.

Even today, the influence of Little Richard's music and peacocking style can be seen. He's inspired guys from Bruno Mars to André 3000, both of whom have said they channeled Little Richard in the way they perform. The rock-and-roll legend broke down barriers and opened the floodgates for other men across all spectrums to feel confident in expressing their identities. Not only was he the founder of an entirely new musical genre, he's still the blueprint for how unstoppable a man can be when he channels his authenticity and dares to live his truth. Little Richard proved that when a man takes that leap, he can become utterly—Tutti Frutti-ly—unstoppable.

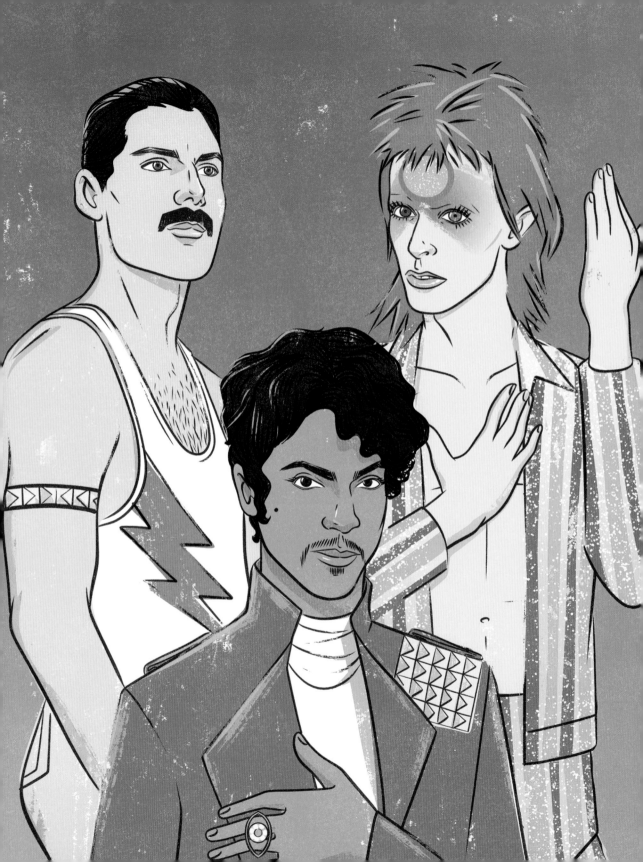

GLAM ROCK

(1 9 7 0 s - 1 9 8 0 s)

Wham glam, thank you, ma'am.

THOUGH THE SIXTIES WERE DEFINED BY MOVEMENTS FOR EQUAL rights, LGBTQIA rights had been left behind. It didn't help that doctors claimed queerness was a mental illness. Any behavior that was outside of the strict binary rulebook—like, say, guys being interested in fashion—was considered "aberrant," a mental illness. Believe it or not, the Beatles had been considered "rebellious" for rocking "effeminate" bowl-cut hairstyles and wearing colorful outfits deemed "flashy."

But bubbling in the British underground were a set of rabble-rousers who were about to paint over heteronormativity in full ROYGBIV. If the 1960s were all about sexual liberation, hippie styles, and sociopolitical revolution, these new revolutionaries took it ten steps further, championing overt, proud, and more fluid displays of gender: a mix of sky-high platform shoes, space-age outfits, astral hair, and, of course, glitter, this was the brand-new age of sexual and individual freedom.

This was glam rock.

In 1971, the curious front man named Marc Bolan of a band called T. Rex debuted on Britain's *Top of the Pops.* With his signature flamingo-colored feather boa, glassy satin shirts, and mosslike velvet trousers, the lead singer floated onstage like an exquisite butterfly, albeit a brawny one. Blush blended into his round cheeks, globs of mascara coated his long lashes, and speckles of glitter shimmered on his face as he flapped his sinewy wings. As Bolan would later explain in an interview for Radio 1, the inspiration came from his wife, June Child, who had a bottle of glitter on her dressing room table. He decided he'd dab it on his face to see if a man could look equally beautiful and ridiculous. The *Independent* would later describe this exact moment as having "permitted a generation of teeny-boppers to begin playing with the idea of androgyny." Bolan's androgyny would later help him come out about his binary-defying sexuality. "[I'm] bisexual," he told *Pop Mirror* magazine in 1975.

T. Rex blew up the charts and paved the way for a wave of glam rockers: Roxy Music, the Sweet, Queen, David Bowie, and, a little later on, Prince. Each was specific with their visual style, defined them as a mix between nostalgic glamour fused with futuristic space-age wonderment, a juxtaposition of revealing, outré, and joyous fashion and makeup with muscular bodies.

....

WHILE BOLAN MAY HAVE OPENED THE DOOR TO GLAM SENSI-bilities, Bowie opened the floodgates, catapulting the genre and its visual representations into the mainstream. Bowie's thoughtful looks would make him an instant sartorial idol. His distinct look was a combination of references that seemed incompatible, but somehow worked: from Kabuki makeup (see "Drag Queens: A Herstory" on page 135) to Marlene Dietrich's poses, combined with the humor and satire of Dada art. Who could forget his fire engine–red hair and blue-and-red lightning bolt on the cover of *Aladdin Sane*? Or the electric blue eyeshadow and icy skin tone in "Life on Mars"? Unparalleled as a musician, Bowie was also unmatched in his artistry. He was also very matter-of-fact with his gay identity, proudly admitting: "Always have been"—though he'd eventually go on to marry two women, including the model Iman.

....

FROM THE START, QUEEN FRONT MAN FREDDIE MERCURY HAD his signature shaggy mullet cut and eyeliner. He'd graduate to more daring looks. In one performance, Mercury powdered his face white, used blush and rouge, while sporting a Japanese samurai robe. He wielded his mic like a sword onstage, pretending he was a warrior. In 1974, he'd enlist a fashion designer named Zandra Rhodes to create custom outfits for him. One was an unforgettable off-white accordion-pleated blouse, inspired by a wedding dress. When he performed during Queen II's era, he'd rock it onstage, accessorized by black-painted nails and eyelids drawn with liner and elongated winged tips. His taut body and open display of thick body hair contrasted with the short shorts, spandex bodysuits, and leotards he'd wear. It was a perfect balance of masculine body and feminine presentation. It was difficult not to be seduced by Mercury, who used his aesthetics and sexuality as deliberate marketing tools. And he was "gay as a daffodil, my dear!" as he'd say in an interview.

While so many celebrities would shy away from these questions, none of these three glam rockers did. While coming out is an often difficult time for many male stars, even today, Bolan, Bowie, and Mercury were unprecedented—at the peak of their careers, all three came out as queer.

At a time when Western culture was still at odds with LGBTQIA identities, the way glam rockers interwove art and identity shone a light into what it meant to be queer—the understanding that each individual's identity could be messy, could be a little of this and a little of that, and that any combination and iteration of expression deserved to take up space. Glam rock and its stars did more than inspire one group of people, though—the genre pushed everyone to come out, let loose, and, even if just for the course of a single song, became who they wanted to be.

AND THEN CAME PRINCE

At his peak, Prince's presence on Earth was so ubiquitous, everyone breathed him in like lavender-scented oxygen (he was notorious for being spritzed in the floral fragrance). And his iteration of glam rock would change the course of music history.

Prince didn't only *exude* sex—he *was* sex. With doe eyes thick with kohl eyeliner, a resplendent complexion accessorized by a beauty mark on his cheek, and a mustache that was carefully groomed into thin shapes that spelled mischief, he could hypnotize with a single glance. His career and performances would provide a *purple*-print for how to challenge stereotypes of what a man—and in particular, a Black man—could be.

By 1978, the charts were crowded with white, cisgendered artists: the Bee Gees, Fleetwood Mac, the Rolling Stones, Billy Joel—these were alt-rockers who had pop sensibilities and more or less looked the same. When Prince dropped his funky and assertively sexual single "Soft and Wet," he busted the doors open, flushing cheeks in the process.

In his music video for "Wanna Be Your Lover," audiences felt the full power of Prince's sensuality. The heat emitted from screens to bodies with every thrash of Prince's hips, every swing of his pelvis. With luscious long locks, a hint of red eye shadow, a single hoop earring, tight jeans, and a shirt revealing a bare chest with thick body hair, he channeled the previous decades' glam rock and Little Richard.

The young artist pushed the boundaries of acceptable displays of sexuality even further for his third album, *Dirty Mind,* with cover art of him wearing nothing but tight black underwear and a leather jacket. Prince's major single "Controversy" taunted his naysayers: "I just can't believe all the things people say / Am I black or white, am I straight or gay?" But it would be *Purple Rain* that solidified Prince in American pop culture—he not only became the number one–selling artist, he became the government's public enemy as well.

In a movement led by Tipper Gore—wife of then senator/now former vice president Al Gore, and an Ultimate Karen—the establishment was out to take the king down. "Darling Nikki," in which Prince sings about female masturbation and sexuality, had Gore enraged. But Prince took it in stride. He famously said, "I don't really care so much what people say about me because it usually is a reflection of who they are." He had more important matters to tend to. That year, he not only released *Purple Rain* the album, but the major motion picture as well. The movie would become a box office hit, and would eventually win him an Oscar and a Golden Globe. "Ultimately, all music is and can be inspirational," he later said, as if addressing all the Karens of the world. "That's why it's so important to let your gift be guided by something really clear."

In April 2016, Prince passed away. In his later years, Prince was as vibrant, prolific, and musically gifted as ever. In the months leading up to his death, Prince still toured, playing sold-out venues, and worked on a book, *The Beautiful Ones,* celebrating his Black community.

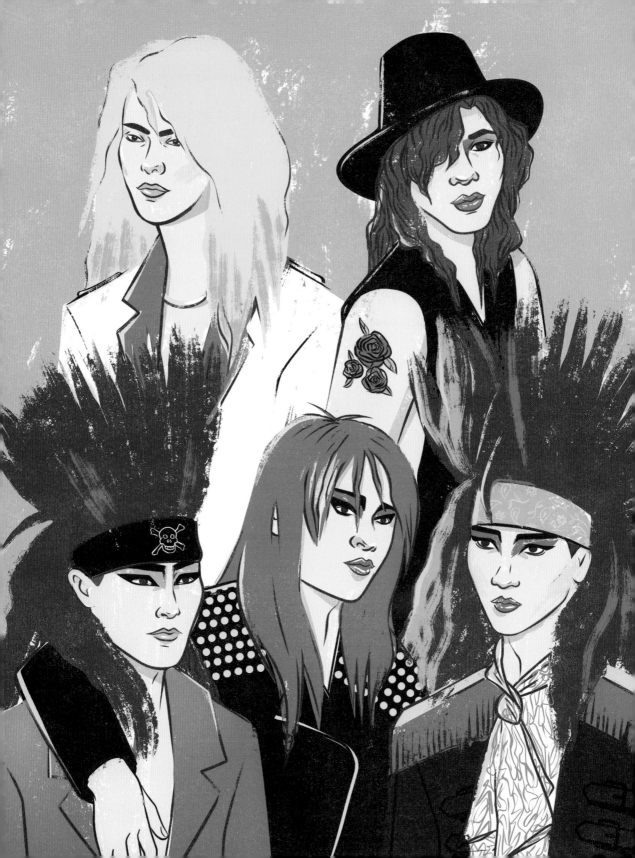

VISUAL KEI

(1 9 8 0 s -)

TW: SUICIDE

AS GLAM ROCK WAS TAKING OVER EUROPE IN THE 1970s, ITS American cousin, glam metal, was thrashing its way across America's West Coast. If glam rock was about adopting androgyny and fluid sexuality, the 1980s went back to promoting heterosexuality and hypermasculinity, albeit through wild hair and crass makeup. The new wave of punk, rock and roll fused into hostile heavy metal: bands like Mötley Crüe, Twisted Sister, Def Leppard, and Bon Jovi became America's politically rebellious new sex symbols, wreaking havoc until the early 1990s.

Halfway around the world in Japan, however, a burgeoning subculture was fusing glam rock and metal and making it local. The marriage between the two brought American metal sound and its antiestablishment nature together with British gender-bending aesthetics. But Japanese artists also added a sprinkle of gothic darkness to create a bold new movement known as "visual *kei*." Japan's own version also embraced hyperfemininity in the form of highly stylized face makeup, dainty women's clothing—from dresses to lacy tights—and over-the-top, intricate hair. The adoption of visual kei would be in direct opposition to Japan's growing capitalistic culture.

As most Asian countries were thrust into economic turmoil, many stricken by poverty and the aftereffects of colonization, Japan emerged as one of the strongest nations in the world. The 1960s, '70s, and '80s were a golden time for the Land of the Rising Sun. The country made an impressive transformation in a matter of a few decades from being labeled an international pariah from its imperialist past and moving forward to become one of the greatest economies in the world. But it came at a cost. To achieve this near-impossible economic feat, Japan enforced a work culture that promoted high efficiency, conformity, and homogeneity. In turn, creatives were shunned and considered as outliers of a productive society.

Of course, everything changed when Japan realized creativity could be capitalized en mass, and the financial impact of soft power—think manga and anime, Nintendo. Music, and visual kei, would become the next largest export.

Formed in the underground scene in the early 1980s, the band X Japan wrote "Psychedelic Violence Crime of Visual Shock" on the cover of their second album, *Blue Blood.* The inscription described freedom of expression that would "shock" from the visual representations of its band members. "Visual shock" was then shortened to "visual-kei." Rather than describing a music genre, visual kei was more about a strong and outlandish aesthetic used to provoke a visceral reaction.

Indeed, the early days of X Japan and visual kei were frightening in their more zealous use of beauty: looks included gargantuan manes that were even bigger than those sported by American hair metal bands, blown out in a multitude of colors. Other styles included large mohawks, with huge spikes that stood two feet into the air. Their makeup was gothic, globs of white foundation, eyes painted with heavy eyeshadows and liners, lips painted in black. "That was the crime of visual shock," said Yoshiki, one of the band members, in an interview in the documentary *We Are X.* "We also wanted to mess up people's minds through music. That's why it's psychedelic violence."

Yoshiki's own life experiences were authentic to the band's message. When the leader of the band was only ten years old, he stumbled onto his father's dead body. "I was very angry and sad. I was only doing classical music," he recalled. "Then I found out about rock. I could scream and break things. I became a rebel." The angst and pain funneled into loud, shrieking music that would be one of the first examples of heavy metal in East Asia. As the documentary's director, Stephen Kijak, stated: "That starts to fuck with society. They realize, 'Oh, we actually have permission to scream and dye our hair and be different and break down barriers.'"

Japanese men have historically explored beyond the boundaries of the binary. Men like the Kabuki, theater performers who adeptly played female roles and wowed Japan's elite, held strong cultural cache, or the *bishonen,* literally translated to "pretty boys" (see page 135 for more on the Edo period). Visual kei, however, promoted hyperfemininity—radically, loudly, and with the intent to aggress.

X Japan and its visual kei movement had a profound effect on youth culture, despite its critics. "A lot of rock people hate us because we are playing super heavy, really fast music, dressed like an anime character, people were like, what are you guys doing?" Yoshiki said in an interview with *Loudwire.* "We didn't care." The popularity of X Japan allowed other bands like Buck-Tick, D'erlanger, and Color, among others, to further push the visual kei movement into the mainstream.

X Japan would slowly make its way around the world, creating an international following. In 2007, J-rock and visual kei held a major event in Los Angeles, performing to American fanfare. The aesthetic has become so popular in places like Germany that there were publications dedicated to visual kei's artistry, history, and fixtures. The country even birthed its own visual kei–inspired acts like of Cinema Bizarre and Tokio Hotel.

Once in the mainstream, bands like Alice Nine (A9) and Dir En Grey and solo acts like Miyavi became household names. The newer acts have taken visual kei's dark roots and translated the movement into something more modern, and more accessible, adopting anime or cosplay references. Today's visual kei stars have largely abandoned goth for more optimistic, joyful colors, shinier fabrics, and makeup and hair that mimic manga characters.

Of course, this hasn't sat well with visual kei's founding fathers. They've since criticized the newer generation for taking their individuality and making it too palatable and imitable in the mainstream, defeating the purpose of the movement's beginnings. While this may be true, one might argue that this is a good thing: today's Japanese youth culture has normalized makeup and beauty, regardless of gender identity, as a way to express individuality. Visual kei paved the way for Japan's many other subcultures—including Lolita and *gyaru,* among others—to thrive, giving future generation options to be as loud, colorful, brash, or gothic as they want to be. The fact that Tokyo and its Harajuku district are internationally recognized today as one of the most expressive places on Earth has everything to do with visual kei.

The fact that Tokyo and its Harajuku district are internationally recognized today as one of the most expressive places on Earth has everything to do with visual kei.

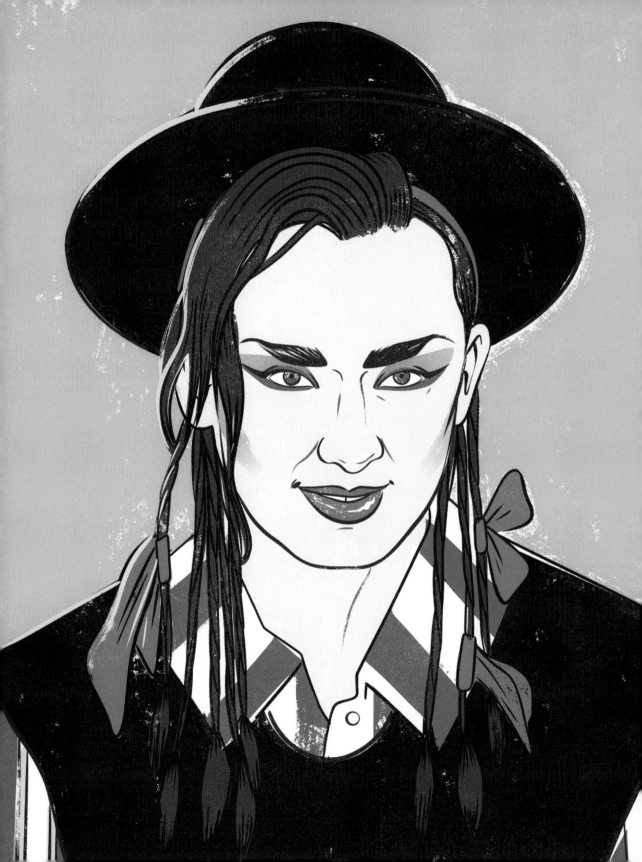

BOY GEORGE

(1 9 6 1 -)

President of the Culture Club.

EARLY INTERVIEWS OF BOY GEORGE ARE NOT ONLY EXCRUCIATING, they're dehumanizing.

He'd made his debut stateside in 1983. Culture Club had just released "Karma Chameleon," and was number two on the Top 100 charts, joining the ranks of many other artists from the UK who had come over as part of the Second British Invasion. But while his peers—the likes of Duran Duran, Def Leppard, and Billy Idol—were gaining recognition for their music, when it came to Boy George, all people wanted to talk about was his style.

His first appearance on *Late Show with David Letterman,* for instance, had Letterman fixated on his aesthetics, and the host failed to mention that "Do You Really Want to Hurt Me" was the hottest record that year.

"Are people puzzled by the way you look?" Letterman asked.

"How long have you been appearing this way?"

"You appear really different."

Boy George, then just twenty-two years old, was sporting a printed yellow cassock. An oversize bowler hovers on top of his braids, and as he bats his long, mascara-globbed lashes, his winged eyeliner reveals icy blue eyes. He's visibly uncomfortable, but still answers every question with grace and confidence.

"People are really boring on the streets," he replies. "I didn't want to be another person with a big nose. I wanted to be a person with a big nose and style."

Later in the interview, with the audience heckling him, Letterman takes it a bit further, trying to out the singer on his show. "You're obviously . . ." he infers of Boy George's possible homosexuality.

"Beautiful," George answers.

On *The Phil Donahue Show* later that year, thirty minutes are dedicated to allowing an all-white, suburban Chicago audience to have a free-for-all with their questions. Boy George listens intently, sporting an oversize electric blue blazer, his face painted gold like a Sphynx, his lips blue, with fiery red hair.

"Why do you dress up like a woman?" an audience member asks.

"Why do you look so weird?" asks another.

"People can't get beyond the way you look."

Johnny Carson would defend these critics later on *The Tonight Show,* saying, "You can't blame them for asking those questions, you *are* rather controversial."

At that point, Boy George was squeaky clean, focused on music, and known for good behavior. The only marginally shocking thing about him was that he was a rock star who didn't trash his hotel rooms.

Long before he'd been subjugated by ignorant American talk show hosts, he'd been dressing up in colorful outfits for years in London. "It was all Bowie's fault," he'd later recall, thinking of how he'd color his hair blue using ink from a pen.

Born George Alan O'Dowd, he was the second of five children. His father ran a boxing club and his mother was a seamstress. When he decided to begin experimenting with his appearance, his parents didn't think much of it. "They never objected," he once told the *Washington Post.* "When I used to come home dressed up, my dad used to roll his eyes in the air and make jokes, but he never really took much notice." He came out to his parents, with his mother acknowledging his sexuality by buying him the Rod Stewart record "The Killing of Georgie." One of its lyrics: "Georgie boy was gay I guess."

He took his self-expression and confidence to school, where he'd be expelled at fifteen for showing up with orange hair. While the other students and teachers may have considered him a rebel, on the streets of Central London, he was gaining acceptance as a part of the

New Romantic movement, a pop culture phenomenon emphasizing over-the-top dress and animated makeup in rejection of the punk movement.

The movement was incubated at the Blitz, a club where Boy George worked in coat check. The venue was the hottest underground party in town and the door was kept tight. Only those with over-the-top outfits, the most unique beauty looks—heavy eyeshadow, painted nails, dark lipstick, and more—were allowed in. The club was so exclusive, even rocker Mick Jagger was turned away.

While working there, Boy George's sense of style caught the attention of Malcolm McLaren, the former manager of the Sex Pistols. Boy was asked to join a group McLaren was working with called Bow Wow Wow, and he was given the stage name Lieutenant Lush. He eventually clashed with the band members and quit, then went off to create his own band with musicians Mikey Craig, Roy Hay, and Jon Moss. Moss, the drummer, would become George's lover, and the subject of many of the songs George would write.

After their world debut on the popular British show *Top of the Pops,* thousands of viewers wrote in, asking if the lead singer was male or female. During the performance, a youthful Boy George could pass as either. His plump face is contoured to accentuate his cheekbones. His eyebrows are shaped like minnows, thicker at the front and thinner at the tail end, his hooded eyes painted with ash-gray shadow. A deep pink blush paints his cheeks, which match the color used on his thick lips. To top it off, he wears his hair in long braids, tied with dozens of white ribbons. He looks spritely, cool, effortless. *Do you really want to hurt me,* he sings, in a rich, sonorous tenor range.

But the New Romantics hadn't crossed the pond—when Boy George did, the American mainstream found him to be *too* androgynous. Gender nonbinary was not yet a term in most Americans' vocabularies. But it was too late—by the time he arrived, they'd already been taken by the beautiful voice and hot track they'd heard on the radio.

The band became the first British group since the Beatles to have three top-ten songs on their debut album. But with success came murmurs about his sexuality. The American press were more ruthless than the British, and wanted Boy George to admit his identity. He often deflected these questions, stating that he preferred thinking about tea.

Then came Joan Rivers. "Do you prefer men or women?" she asked bluntly in a 1983 taping of her show. "Oh, both," a visibly uncomfortable Boy George said. He'd later tell *Spin* magazine in 1989 that he lamented ever coming out. "When we first went to America they thought I was a cute oddity," he said. "That was before they knew that I was gay. Now they know. I think I'm suffering for it now."

In 1986, Boy George was arrested for heroin possession. The press reveled in the moment. The *Washington Post* wrote: "Police drug investigators this morning ended a two-day search for Boy George, the 25-year-old 'gender-bender' pop star whose heavy makeup and female attire has alarmed parents and entranced young record buyers, after his recording company announced he was under medical treatment." Parents and politicians from America to Britain felt like this would be the end of George's career. "It is so unfortunate that somebody like Boy George should set a very bad example to youth," said Baroness Trumpington, a member of the British Conservative Party.

But the youths would disagree, and they cherished his authenticity, the way his sensual ambiguity issued a direct challenge to glam rock and heavy metal hypersexuality. From his youth to now, the artist has consistently expressed himself through his silver tongue and golden makeup, his makeup and beauty acting as armor when words were insufficient, or too much. While it may have been protective for him then, his style and his work have led the charge in breaking down boundaries of expression today.

WHILE IT MAY HAVE BEEN PROTECTIVE for HIM THEN, HIS STYLE and HIS WORK HAVE LED the CHARGE in BREAKING DOWN BOUNDARIES of EXPRESSION TODAY.

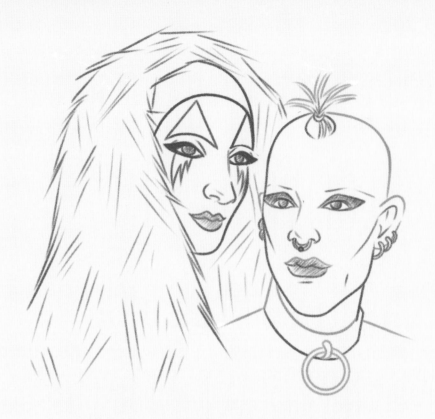

CLUB KIDS

(1980s)

Fabulous misfits.

IT'S TWO A.M., AND HUNDREDS OF SWEATY BODIES ARE PRESSED against each other, creating a feverish, brackish fog. A blaring trance beat reverberates as neon lights draw lines on painted faces. Their mouths agape in ecstasy, mascara drizzling down their melted faces, they strut, twirl, and *work* as if they're getting paid.

These are the Club Kids, a collective of underground queer creatives, artists, and performers, and this is the Limelight in New York City, an Episcopal church turned nightclub, a mecca for pariahs and misfits alike.

Flaunting exaggerated, original, DIY looks, Club Kids are all about shock value and attention. Club Kids feed off being photographed, the buzz they receive from local and national press. It's the late '80s, and they're fighting against the media, and American culture as a whole, which has villainized the LGBTQIA community amid the AIDS crisis. And they're doing it through iconic parties.

....

The Club Kids began with a handful of New York City's biggest nightlife fixtures. These included artist Walt Cassidy, model Amanda Lepore, and designer Richie Rich, among many others. Typical looks include bright hair, body piercings, big wigs, towering heels, exaggerated accessories, patent leather. Makeup is fantastical: pencil-thin eyebrows, long wispy lashes, stark white face paint popping with bright eyeshadows and blushes, overdrawn lipstick, and raccoon eyeliner.

Tonight, like any other weeknight, these partygoers have flocked to the bumping, thumping Limelight, which sits at the corner of Twentieth Street and Sixth Avenue in New York's Chelsea neighborhood. A line of young people winds around the block, some new, some old—all desperate for validation in the form of entry. Already inside are the Club Kid elite, which would expand to include RuPaul, designer Patricia Field, and DJ Keoki, among others. "It felt like walking through the gates of heaven," Walt Cassidy, who attended his first Club Kid party at nineteen, will later recall. "The doors opened and every possibility was open to me." Being a Club Kid means that you have to *serve* original looks that were intentional in blurring gender and sexuality norms, looks that were anti-mainstream. The more your look would make older generations shake, the better.

In a few years, Club Kids would get the attention they craved for all their over-the-top antics—they'd shock television airwaves when they were invited on talk shows like *Geraldo,* or covered in op-eds and articles in national papers. Parents everywhere would be frightened for their children's futures. They began to become commercial properties, inspiring mass music, fashion, beauty, film, and television. Later, musicians like Elton John, designers like Jean Paul Gaultier, and photographers like David LaChapelle would use Club Kid lifestyle as a source of inspiration.

At the beginning of the 1990s, the Club Kids dissolved, in part due to the murder of one member by one of their leaders. Rumors of violence throughout the community led to the government stepping in. With backlash from the general public and Mayor Rudy Giuliani's "Quality of Life" crackdown on the city's many clubs, the Club Kids had fewer places to gather and eventually dispersed into the pages of history. While they were the last influencers of the analog era, their influence still pervades culture, today. We can turn to fashion to see just how club kids have inspired generations from the likes of Lady Gaga, who credits club kids for her own style; high-end brands from Gucci to Opening Ceremony, which both frequently take nods from '90s New York City swagger for its collections; to makeup artists like Pat McGrath who study the youth of the era's beauty looks for a modern-day audience. In infiltrating national media with their brilliant looks, gender nonconforming aesthetics, fearless sexuality, their time in the limelight kept the door propped open for proceeding generations to imagine more possibilities than what the mainstream lens wants us to see. To be remembered is exactly how they would have wanted it.

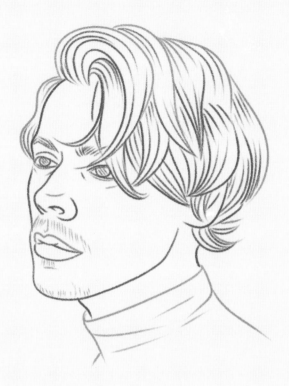

HARRY STYLES

(1 9 9 4 -)

The metamorphosis of a teen idol.

MASCULINITY AS A CONSTRUCT: DOES IT FLOW IN ONE DIREC-tion, or does it swerve on both sides of the binary, moving in arbitrary squiggles, dancing along thick, dotted lines? It's a question that Harry Styles, the former boy band wunderkind, seems to be working through ever since he began warping around the globe as one-fifth of the group One Direction.

While One Direction is no more, from its inception Harry had stood out for his rambunctious behavior, cheeky charm, and sweet demeanor. While he played the part of a teen idol like a dream, behind that handsome veneer—those dimpled cheeks, long-lashed eyes, devious smile—was someone who was processing more complex expressions of identity. In 2014 fans were delighted to get a glimpse of this: when an interviewer from a talk show asked him and his bandmate Liam Payne what they looked for in a lover, his answer left tongues wagging. "Female," Liam said snarkily. "That's an important trait." Styles, on the other hand, shook his head, almost bored with his bandmate's answer. "Not that important," he replied matter-of-factly, looking at the ground. The camera pans to Payne, who sinks himself into his seat. His cheeks are red—he seems confused or uncomfortable, or both. Whether he knew it then or not, Styles was on the verge of leading music into a more nonbinary future.

The following year at the 2015 American Music Awards, most of One Direction hit the red carpet in coordinated muted gray suits and oxfords. Meanwhile, Styles—his mane newly grown out—sported a Gucci suit in a delicious black wallpaper floral pattern on a cream background. His trousers were flared, a nod to '70s bell-bottoms, at this point still considered a feminine sartorial choice. The daring look was almost *too* much for the world to handle. The transition from masc-presenting heartthrob to risk-taking fashionista was a shock to the senses. "What was Harry Styles thinking?" wrote one publication in New Zealand. "Harry Styles's AMA suit looks like everybody's bedspread," wrote *Cosmopolitan.* But Harry was undeterred. He was on a journey, critics be damned. "I had never really done flares before and it was really fun," he later recalled in an interview with *Dazed* magazine in 2017. "I just kind of started wearing more and more of it, and at the same time just becoming a lot more comfortable in myself."

He left 1D that year. As a newly freed solo artist, Styles delved into not only discovering what his individual voice would be, but also his sense of self. His eponymous first album, released in 2017, focused on identity and authenticity. The lead single, "Sign of the Times," spoke to fighting to live in your truth, being open to varying identities, of being yourself and being beautiful. In photos accompanying an interview with *Rolling Stone* just before the album's release, Styles sits in the back seat of a car, sporting a black floral jacquard suit with a bright pink satin pussy-bow blouse. His eyes smolder. He looks vulnerable, elegant.

"I don't think people are still looking for this gender differentiation," he later explained to *L'Officiel.* "Even if the masculine and feminine exist, their limits are the subject of a game. We no longer need to be this or that . . . and it gives rise to great freedom. It's stimulating." At 2018's Met Gala, he goes further toward nonconformity, sporting a sheer, nipple-grazing Gucci one-piece, a single dangling pearl earring, with black and white nails accentuating his overall look.

"What women wear. What men wear. For me it's not a question of that," he explained to the *Guardian*. "If I see a nice shirt and get told, 'But it's for ladies.' I think: 'Okaaaay? Doesn't make me want to wear it less though.' I think the moment you feel more comfortable with yourself, it all becomes a lot easier."

With the release of his second album, 2019's *Fine Line,* Styles became even more deliberate with the details, with beauty. This time, instead of flaunting a more colorful sense of style, he began painting his nails with bright hues, adding shapes: fruit, smiley faces, flowers, and more. Nail art soon became as synonymous with Harry as his thick, wavy brunette hair. In an editorial for 2020's *Beauty Papers,* he's photographed posing in nothing but fishnet stockings. His face is full of makeup, with blush, eyes lined in black, eyelids stroked with eyeshadow, his lips painted a rosy pink. He appears confident and free—like he has full agency of his body, his face, his prettiness. This is the Harry Styles he'd been working toward.

Years later, ex-bandmate Payne is asked about Harry's striking transformation. For Payne, witnessing Harry's metamorphosis hasn't been easy. "There's so much mystery around who he's kind of become," he admitted to *The Face*. "I was actually genuinely looking at some pictures of him the other day, and I just thought, 'I don't know what more I'd say to him.'" Everything has changed, but nothing has changed. He's still the same Harry that Payne, fans, and critics observed throughout his teenage years and on into his adulthood. It's just that at this time, he's metamorphosed and stretched out vibrant new wings, free to stretch, flutter, and explore this brand-new world.

"We no longer need to be this or that . . . and it gives rise to great freedom."

— HARRY STYLES

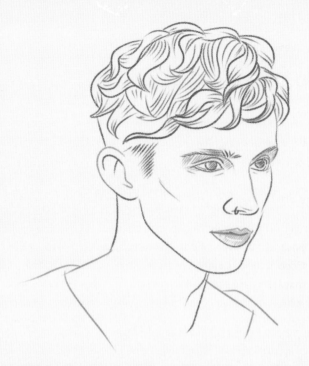

TROYE SIVAN

(1 9 9 5 -)

A twinkle in time.

"I THINK 2012 ME WOULD HAVE BEEN REALLY SCARED OF 2018 me," the artist named Troye Sivan once tweeted. "Too gay."

It's hard to imagine that the Australian pop sensation would have ever been anything less than fearless when it comes to his identity. Are we talking about the same South Africa–born singer, who's unapologetic when it comes to queer expression—especially as it relates to beauty? In his video for "Bloom," a coming-of-age anthem all about losing your anal virginity, Troye serves effortless glamour with wet, slicked-back platinum blond hair, lips painted fire engine red, eyelids gleaming with bright bubblegum pink eyeshadow. In his campaigns for Glossier Play and MAC Cosmetics, he oozes sensuality, a full face of glamour painted on him like a second skin. And on red carpets from the Met Gala to stages across the world,

Troye smirks coyly at every camera knowing exactly how his highlighter pops with every flash.

Though he's certainly on his way to joining the ranks of the iconoclastic musicians who paved a beautiful path before him—among them Little Richard, Prince, Bowie, and Boy George,—like them, he first had to reckon with his biggest critic: himself.

Back when he was a teenager growing up in Perth, a coastal city in Australia, Troye Sivan Mellet was an imaginative boy. As yet makeup-free, he first entered the public eye as Australia's biggest YouTuber, with millions of subscribers tuning in to watch him sing and perform. Using the platform as a launchpad, he began landing parts in Hollywood, playing a young Wolverine in *X-Men Origins: Wolverine,* while also releasing original music.

Then in 2013, he posted a video of him coming out, three years after he told his family he was gay. He'd practiced how he'd do it, watching other coming out videos, nervous about the repercussions against his nascent career. Instead, that same year, Capitol Records signed him to their label, where he joined other singers like Sam Smith. With newfound fame and an international platform, Troye began to blossom into a beauty boy. First to change was his hair, which he bleached platinum blond. On his first big performance on NBC's *Saturday Night Live,* his face has a bit of blush, with highlighter on his cheekbones and forehead. When he started appearing on magazine covers, from *Wonderland* to *Teen Vogue* to *VMan* and many others, it was apparent that his aesthetics were becoming more fluid, gender-bending. In his *Wonderland* spread, he sports a feminine blush cami with thin spaghetti straps hanging over his body. In *Attitude* magazine, his eyes are drawn in, thick with eyeliner and mascara.

And so it's surprising that Troye still wasn't completely confident in beautifying, outside of the looks and makeup stylists were putting him in for editorials. "Coming out as gay is one thing," he once told *Harper's Bazaar.* "And then coming out as the person you want to be is a whole other separate journey. Although I came out as gay to my family, there was still a lot I hid: the way I wanted to move, dress, speak."

And then he shot the video for "Bloom." He recalled being a bit nervous on set, asking himself if the colorful beauty looks were really him. "Does this feel real to me? Does this feel genuine to me?" Of course, eventually trying on the looks and scrutinizing himself in the mirror made it all feel natural. "Why stop yourself?" he remembers asking himself. "Who are you stopping yourself for? I feel like I'm like super publicly gay, but that self-doubt, that's part of the journey for me. It's about pushing through that."

Today, Troye is one of Gen Z's best known faces, working as an ambassador for major beauty brands and proudly showing off his beauty and skincare routine for all the world to see in *Vogue.* A long way away from the young Australian boy who was once afraid to be too outwardly expressive and "gay," today's Troye has pushed further past the boundaries than 2012 Troye would have even imagined.

HAIR TO DYE FOR

Everything you need to know before you bleach your hair.

Fans may be waiting with bated breath for Jimin's next hair color reveal, but hair dyeing isn't a new phenomenon. In fact, dyeing goes all the way back to ancient Egypt, where wigs were dyed black, red, blue, green, or gold with henna—a potent and long-lasting ingredient that stained anything in touched. The Greeks and Romans also used henna, a natural dye, but used the chemicals lead oxide and calcium hydroxide in dyes as well (which would prove to be *way* too harsh for skin).

While some dyed their hair to remove grays, others bleached their coifs as a requirement. During the earlier years of the Roman Empire, sex workers were forced to lighten their hair to proclaim their profession. Some wore wigs colored with dyes made from nuts, plants, and other natural ingredients, mixed with chemicals. By the 1700s, hair coloring was becoming en vogue in Europe, and many people would put lye in their hair and sit in the sun to bleach it. Whatever the process, hair bleaching has never been easy. The process of bleaching forcibly removes melanin from your hair and the darker the hair, the more melanin, and the more difficult it is to bleach and dye.

To enlighten us on the hair bleaching process, we asked go-to Hollywood hair colorist Rita Hazan for all the *ends* and outs. Rita has worked with everyone—Beyoncé, Mariah Carey, Jennifer Lopez, Jessica Simpson, and *every* other musical icon—and is known in particular for getting tresses colored into her signature honey blond tones. Here's what you need to know before and after getting your hair dyed.

1. COLOR ME MINE.

Before you get the color of your dreams, you need to manifest it first. This comes in the form of finding a capable hairstylist. Consulting with them on which colors would be best for you is much better than bringing in photos from social media. "Instagram isn't always a great reference because there are many filters involved," Rita says. "I think it's always better to ask people in real life and consult with a colorist."

2. NO DYE BUT TODAY.

There are three types of hair coloring:

Permanent color to cover grays or lighten hair without bleach.

Semi/demi-permanent darker color. The dye is ammonia-free and doesn't penetrate hair strands, and the color washes out. "Basically you can think of this as a stain and only darkens the hair," says Rita.

Bleach will lighten your hair to platinum, which is the harshest of all colors. "It will lighten your hair to a yellow color. Then you'll have to tone/color it to soften it up and make it more blond/ash/beige/platinum," Rita explains.

3. LIFE'S A BLEACH.

Seriously, dyeing your hair takes a long time, especially if you need to bleach first. It could take an entire day depending on how thick, long, or dark your hair is. "If you hair is black you will want to take your time and bleach it in stages so you don't damage your hair too much and have a catastrophe," Rita says. "If your hair is virgin or has been colored, you can do it in one session." Ultimately, everyone is different, and you have to make sure you are not in a rush.

4. BURN, BABY, BURN.

From tingling sensations to full-out burning—bleaching isn't a game. While celebrities come out on the red carpets with dazzling new shades, what isn't shown are the hours of tears or downright pain they've endured. "The burn depends on your sensitivity and how long the bleach is on your scalp," Rita says. "If your hair is very dark, you have to use a bleach that is very strong, and it can burn your scalp, but once you wash it off, it should calm down immediately."

5. AFTERCARE IS ABSOLUTE CARE.

After you've survived the bleaching and dyeing process, you have to condition your hair—a lot. "It's dehydrated and somewhat damaged from being bleached, so make sure to hydrate and condition your hair and use products for color-treated hair," Rita says. These include hair masks, deep conditioners, hair oils to replenish, and hair essences to put vitamins back in. The key is being gentle—your hair's been through hell and back. For longer-lasting lightened tresses, try using a purple shampoo to counteract any yellow or orange tones that may appear as your toner or dye fades as well. But do know that it's inevitable that your hair will turn yellow, and your roots will grow out in no time, which means you'll have to go back for a refresh or choose another color altogether.

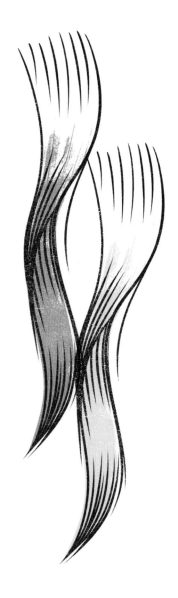

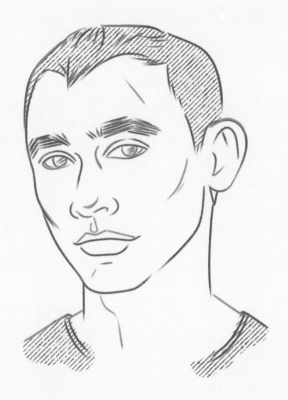

NICOLA
FORMICHETTI

(1 9 7 7 -)

*How Lady Gaga's stylist went from college
dropout to building his own brand.*

IN THE WORLD OF FASHION, THERE ARE ONLY A HANDFUL OF stylists who are respected and labeled as modern-day icons. Among them is Nicola Formichetti, a stylist who translated his career into becoming a creative director and then to founding his own brand, Nicopanda. Along the way, Nicola's overseen brand direction for well-known companies like Uniqlo, Diesel, Mugler, and most recently Lady Gaga's first beauty brand, Haus Laboratories.

This last comes as no surprise. After all, Nicola's been the creative behind Lady Gaga's style from the beginning of her career, from her infamous 2010 MTV Video Music Awards meat dress to the *egg* she was carried in at the 2011 Grammys to all the facial prosthetics she's used and her latest looks in the era of *Chromatica*. We caught up with the star to talk about his early days as a London club kid, growing up biracial in Japan and Italy, and how he came to find success through embracing his authenticity.

....

I NEVER THOUGHT THAT I FIT IN ANYWHERE. I HATED MYSELF when I was little because when we were in Japan I looked different, so I couldn't fit in. I was always trying to make myself look more Asian, trying to blend in. I used to hate the fact that my dad would talk to me in Italian in Japan. "We're in Japan, don't speak in Italian!" We lived outside of Tokyo in a very small town. My brother and I were the only two foreigners in that city. People would come to visit my school to visit foreigners even though we were half Japanese.

When I went to a boarding school in Italy, there was this sense of "othering" there, too. I didn't look Italian, so people thought I was Asian there, and I didn't fit in. At that time I started to own my individuality through fashion and music. I began reading magazines—the Japanese ones, especially. It's really interesting because they had a full page on how to pluck your eyebrows in a men's magazine. I was thirteen, learning how to pluck my eyebrows and wash my face, how to get rid of pimples. It was in my teenage years that I learned more about how to dress up and find my sexuality and learned it's okay to express yourself with beauty and fashion. That's when I started learning that maybe it's cool to be different. Slowly, I started to get my mojo.

I started sneaking into gay clubs when around seventeen. I was really into this red eye look. It was very Alexander McQueen from his shows. It looked like red lipstick around your eyes. I always used to put in one blue eye contact like David Bowie (whose pupil in his left eye was damaged, leaving it permanently discolored) when I would go clubbing. I had a double agent life in high school. I wasn't out and could only be myself when I was outside of the school. During the day people thought I was a good Japanese boy at school and then, at night, a crazy Italian fashion kid. It wasn't until I moved to London when I became really myself. I started seeing people like me in clubs, and it made me go "wow." We were speaking the same language.

At that time it was *i-D* magazine, *The Face,* and *Dazed* magazine that were my bibles. They would feature McQueen, Owen Gaster, very '90s designers who were half club, half high fashion. I was getting noticed because of how I dressed and because of my crazy makeup. I was working at a vintage store and people were like, "That's that kid from that store." One day, *Dazed* asked me to style a photoshoot looking exactly like me. For me, the street and the underground club scene was my school because I didn't go to college. It was the entryway for me, and suddenly, it became a profession I had no idea existed.

I became an assistant editor at *Dazed* and moved my way into becoming the creative director. After ten years I decided to move to New York. I was getting bored and I wanted to do more. People thought I was crazy for leaving this high-positioned job. Going to New York made me feel that same excitement as I did starting out. The differences between the two cities was that in London, it was considered uncool to care about making money. In New York, it was encouraged.

My first gig was for *V Magazine.* The subject of that issue was Lady Gaga. Back then, she was an up-and-coming musician. We met in LA on set and got along really well. She asked me for advice right away: "What do you think I should wear for this thing I'm doing tomorrow," for an Ellen DeGeneres interview. I remember saying to her, "Oh, you should wear this headpiece because that will be interesting when you're talking and this orb [is] moving around your face."

She wore that the next day, and it made news, everywhere. My mind was blown. Normally in a magazine you photograph a model in crazy clothes and then you wait three to four months for it to come out. With her, it was a 3-D experience because I saw my subject moving in what I styled. It was a new sensation for me that I loved. She then asked me what she should do for this live event she was filming in Canada the following week. We started working together.

Gaga and I worked closely for a long time, and our creativity became very spontaneous. We were very good students, studying a lot of history and what was happening in the world. We were also like children, fascinated with a new world. We always used to say we would plan something for a specific project and then on the day of, one minute before it happened, we'd break it, put it upside down, and do something different. That was always our spontaneous process. We were having fun. We were very serious but also not serious at all. That's magic. I call it our golden years. She dominated the fashion, the art, and the music, and it was a fuck-you to everybody.

I was always kind of a backstage person but it was Gaga who pushed me into the limelight. People started wondering who this person was who was working with her. I was known in the industry but not globally. I then received offers to do more projects separate from her. Then I got offered to do Mugler in Paris. This was unheard of for a stylist to take on a fashion house. Gaga was the one who said fucking do it, it would be amazing.

So I left to embark on my own journey having no idea how to do that. Gaga was very encouraging and we transitioned her to Brandon [Maxwell], who was my then assistant. He started taking over all of her stuff. I moved to Paris for a couple of years to become more corporate.

I became less creative when I put a businessman's hat on. I moved on to Diesel and Uniqlo. I was still creative but more in a commercial and business sense. But after almost a decade, I was missing why I went into fashion in the first place. I missed the crazy makeup, fashion, beauty, the avant-garde. That's when I quit everything and moved back to New York and did my own thing. I went back to styling again because I love creating images and moments with people.

As I was doing my own thing, launching Nicopanda (a gender-agnostic apparel brand)—which went on to MAC Cosmetics collaborations—Gaga called me and asked me to work on the Enigma show in Las Vegas. I decided to go to LA again to work with her. I remembered again how amazing it is to work with her. Almost ten years later, we were both different, more mature. I had knowledge on merchandising and all of these other things. It feels like we are now back together again for her *Chromatica* era. It feels like the old days, but at the same time I'm really loving this new era for her. Naturally, I transitioned to helping with Haus Labs, Gaga's first beauty brand, to support her.

Looking back, it's only through me embracing my whole self when the universe opened. Something clicked and I became more comfortable with where I was from; instead of being ashamed of my identity, I realized I was unique. I'm from Japan but I'm also from Italy. When I incorporated that essence into my work, it completely changed. I started being original and confident. There's only one you, and that you is more than enough.

"Looking back, it's only through me embracing my whole self when the universe opened."
—NICOLA FORMICHETTI

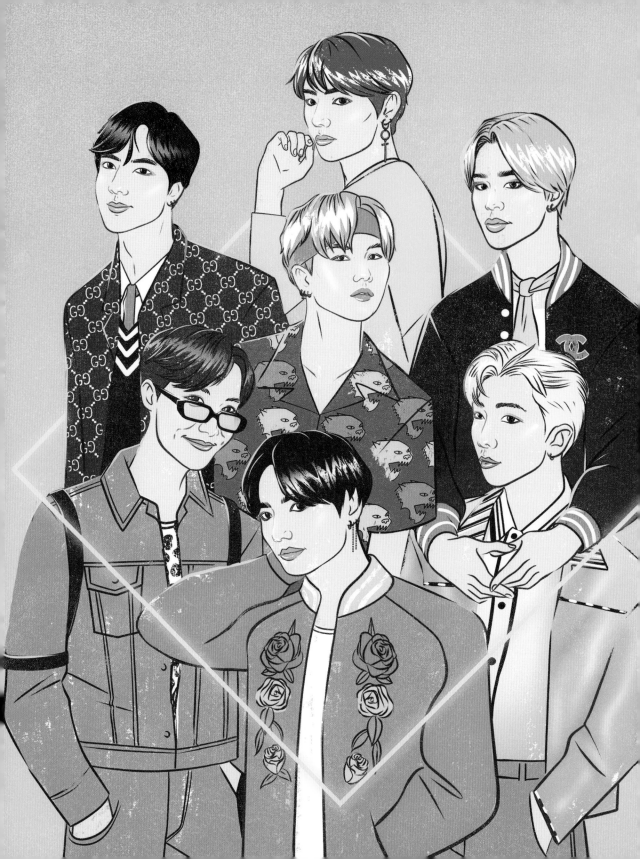

BTS

(2 0 1 0 -)

The greatest boy band—period.

IN 2020, BTS (BANGTAN SONYEONDAN) BECAME THE FIRST South Korean band to make it to number one on the Billboard Hot 100 with their single, "Dynamite," beating out Cardi B and Megan Thee Stallion's "WAP," Harry Styles's "Watermelon Sugar," as well as Drake's "Laugh Now Cry Later." It was historic, as no South Korean music act had achieved such a feat—ever.

But it also wasn't unexpected, as the group had already achieved so much. This is BTS after all, the biggest boy band on record. BTS sold out world stadiums in mere minutes; shattered multiple records, including having the highest number of music video views in 24 hours for their single "Dynamite"; and are tied with the Beatles for most number one albums in a single year (three). For all the acclaim and adoration they've gotten, BTS has also prioritized giving back to their fans and communities—in 2020, the band silently donated $1 million to the Black Lives Matter movement, and they've partnered with UNICEF on "Love Myself," a global youth antiviolence campaign.

This deep empathy for others perhaps stems from the band's own experiences with adversity—after all, BTS was a K-pop group once considered a failure even before they debuted. During their rise, the seven members of BTS faced immense scrutiny and a range of adversities. But what makes BTS so remarkable isn't their music, flashy dance moves, or dewy complexions—rather, it's their ability to connect to their audiences on a human level. Each of the members have been outspoken advocates of mental health, self-love, and self-worth, as well as lending individual support to communities in need, all in a conservative country where these multilayered topics are still considered controversial.

Today, their stories and songs of resilience inspire millions of fans around the world to find the beauty in themselves and become advocates. BTS's fans—the ARMY—resonate with the group's overall message: To conquer the world, you have to love yourself first. To love others, you must confront who you are. Online and off, ARMY spreads messages of love, rallies behind political activism, and donates to causes on BTS's behalf—they might be the most uplifting fandom of any musical artist in the world (in history!).

....

THE FIRST BTS MEMBER RECRUITED FOR THE GROUP IS A K-POP misfit, a rapper named Kim Namjoon (who'd later go by RM), a teen already making a name for himself on the underground hip-hop scene. He's impressive, but doesn't necessarily fit the traditional K-pop aesthetic. His skin tone is deeper, in contrast to Korea's fixation with milky complexions. His eyes are more almond in shape, without double eyelids, which goes against Korean beauty standards at the time.

All of this isn't germane to visionary producer Bang Si-Hyuk of Big Hit Entertainment, and he signs the musical genius on the spot. Bang is on a mission to dismantle the notorious corruption in the K-pop industry, inspire youth, and make change in stifled South Korea—to do so, he isn't leading with what other agencies would be looking for. For him, it's not only raw talent, but empathy—young people who are on the same mission of change.

Years later, Bang and RM convince six other talented teens to join their band of misfits. They include Min Yoongi, a fellow rapper who'll later go by the name Suga, short for "shooting guard," for his love for basketball; Jung Hoseok (J-Hope), a strong dancer who would round out the rapper lineup. The four others include the band's vocalists: Kim Seokjin (Jin), a freshman college student studying acting; Park Jimin, a modern dancer, still in high school; Kim Taehyung (who'd later go by V for "victory"), a singer with an unusual husky voice; and Jeon Jungkook the *maknae* ("youngest"), a shy but charismatic middle schooler. Together, they're the Bangtan Sonyeondan ("Bulletproof Boy Scouts"), aka BTS. The significance of the name: "to block out stereotypes, criticisms, and expectations that aim on adolescents like bullets."

They move into a claustrophobic one-bedroom apartment. Eat, sleep, and train K-pop, dancing and singing for twelve hours a day, balancing school on the side. All the while, they're documenting their fears, hopes, and aspirations on the Twitter account that their agency launches before their debut. Interacting with fans, posting selfies and backstage videos, and showcasing their personalities, they gain a small but active fan base.

When their debut finally arrives in 2013, Bang is running out of funds. The company is on the brink of going under. And it shows. When BTS hits their debut stage, some commenters suggest their look is amateur at best. With baggy outfits that awkwardly hang off their bodies, haircuts that are shaggy, and eyeliner that some say is a bit too dark, they pale in comparison to other established and polished acts. But what they lack in aesthetics, they make up for with immense showmanship. For one, Jimin becomes an instant flirtatious heartthrob, playfully showing off his abs; Jungkook hits high notes with ease; RM owns the stage with his cyphers; J-Hope moves his body with fluidity; Suga slays with his rap verses; Jin's visuals send hearts aflutter; and V's overall singing and dancing make him a super-versatile stage presence.

While other bands at the time sing about unrequited love, BTS is hyperfocused on telling real stories of youth experiences. They write about complex topics ranging from societal pressures on young people, prejudice toward the disenfranchised, and the anxieties that come from growing up in stifling South Korea. But it doesn't quite translate, and their first lead single, "No More Dream," hits the music charts at #124 and falls off quickly afterward.

Though they continue to push through with better performances, elevated outfits, and makeup, they become lost in the sea of competition. Soon enough, television stations begin cutting their performances short, canceling meet-and-greets, and labeling them as failures. To make matters worse, online trolls target the group's members and bully them for their appearance. Other music artists openly criticize them as well. At a roundtable discussion on the state of hip-hop in 2013, an artist berates RM and Suga, accusing them of being fake rappers. He digs at their makeup and sense of style, questioning their sexual and gender identities and arguing that true hip-hop artists must adhere to a specific aesthetic standard. "Doesn't dressing like a girl, wearing makeup, mean you are a girl?" he asks.

The band absorbs the feedback but remains undeterred—they release their next single, "N.O," a song about the unfair and claustrophobic societal pressures on young people, which peaks at #92. They're gaining momentum, and also some attention. They star in SBS MTV's reality show "Rookie King: Channel Bangtan," and the visibility cultivates a slightly larger, robust fan base, who call themselves ARMY (Adorable Representative MC for Youth). In 2015, they find modest success, and hold their first fan meeting with over 3,000 people in attendance. Now, two years into their debut, they shed their hip-hop aesthetic, exploring more of a softer sensibility. Less dark eyeliner, more neutral eyeshadow, spiky hair grown out into bright, colorfully dyed locks. They continue writing songs about youth and anxiety, and begin to discuss depression openly, in spite of taboos, in spite of how stigmatizing it is for an idol group to speak about mental health.

Their third official EP, *The Most Beautiful Moment in Life Pt. I,* becomes their first commercial success, with singles like "I Need U" charting in the top five in Korea, and "Dope" hitting number three on *Billboard*'s World Digital Song Sales chart. But as the band finds some success, they also become targets of renewed online vitriol. They're accused of *sajaegi,* a word that refers to the illegal practice of buying albums in bulk to bolster sales and manipulate the music charts. After months of investigations, BTS is finally cleared. But the experience isn't without extreme emotional turmoil and duress, not to mention embarrassment. As Bang would later lament, "We didn't even have any money if we wanted to do that." Korean fans are perplexed about how a boy band from a little-known record label outside of the Big 3 could have the audacity to succeed.

The next year, the band finally broke through with *The Most Beautiful Moment in Life: Young Forever.* In "Not Today," from the album *You Never Walk Alone,* their lyrics speak to the millions of struggling and disenfranchised South Koreans: "If you can't fly, then run. Today we will survive. If you can't run, then walk. Today we will survive. If you can't walk, then crawl." "Spring Day" hopes for a brighter tomorrow: "The morning will come again. No darkness, no season is eternal." And in "2! 3!," they sing about enduring pain: "Erase all sad memories. Hold each other's hands and smile."

In 2017, the band goes international. With almost half of Twitter now following BTS, the Billboard Music Awards celebrate them as the year's Top Social Artist, beating out mega-artists like Selena Gomez and Justin Bieber. In the live televised awards show, the seven boys walk onstage and shine, beaming to an audience full of artists they've long admired. It's not only validating, but a miracle of sorts—just a few years ago, they were barely scraping by.

But what should have been a moment to shine became yet another instance of immense backlash—an Asian band receiving so much recognition triggers xenophobia, racism, and homophobic tweets about the guys' colorful hair and makeup on a global level. But the band has prepared their entire careers to stand against hate. Channeling their superpowers of focusing on positivity and inspiration, they drop another multiplatinum album, *Love Yourself: Answer;* followed by *Map of the Soul: Persona* and *Map of the Soul: 7,* which would go on to sell over 4 million copies, becoming South Korea's best-selling album ever.

In 2018, BTS is invited to speak at the UN on youth culture. Candidly, precisely, methodically, RM reads a speech that he's written himself.

"Even after making the decision to join BTS, there were a lot of hurdles," RM admits. "Some people might not believe but most people thought we were hopeless. And sometimes, I just wanted to quit. But I think I was very lucky that I didn't give it all up. And I'm sure that I, and we, will keep stumbling and falling like this. No matter who you are, where you're from, your skin color, your gender identity, just speak yourself. Find your name and find your voice by speaking yourself."

BTS is a beacon of hope—while continuing to dominate the charts, they're sending a bigger message: Love can extinguish hate. And ultimately, embracing your self can light up the world—some would say like dynamite.

"NO MATTER WHO YOU ARE, WHERE YOU'RE FROM, YOUR SKIN COLOR, YOUR GENDER IDENTITY... FIND YOUR NAME and FIND YOUR VOICE BY SPEAKING YOURSELF." —RM

KOREAN BOY BEAUTY SECRETS

Influencer Ivan Lam shares how K-beauty changed his life.

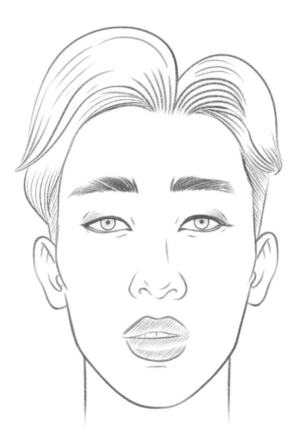

YouTuber and influencer Ivan Lam has amassed hundreds of thousands of followers thanks to his Korean beauty–inspired tutorials. Lam, a proud Malaysian American, is part of a new generation of YouTube beauty gurus who are sharing tips, exchanging cultures, and showing the universality of beauty—in Lam's case, K-beauty. We get the low-down on the best tips Lam's come across, the one thing he always does for gleaming skin, and how to "cheat" your way through to glass skin (a trend in K-beauty where your skin looks translucent like glass) goals. "Dew" the right thing and read on for all his gleaming tips.

Tell me about getting onto YouTube and becoming a social media star—how'd that happen?

It happened quite randomly, actually. My first video was filmed in one of my friends' video sets. She asked if I wanted to put on makeup and I agreed. The world works in such mysterious ways when you say yes. Doors really do open. Nothing happens overnight, of course, but I fell in love with absorbing and sharing my knowledge. Growing up in Malaysia, I rarely found time to think about my own identity. I was really busy studying and going to tuition classes. I always knew that I was different, though, and most of my close friends were females. I grew up being a little bit more overweight than my peers due to stress from school, so I would be really insecure. Malaysia is also quite humid and I grew up with very reactive acne-prone skin. That's definitely one of the reasons I started trying beauty products out. I kept uploading videos on skincare and makeup—and here I am.

Can you give us insights into Korean beauty and how you stumbled upon it? What was the first product that changed your life?

I think in Asia skincare in general plays a huge role in daily life. Clean, flawless skin was always the standard, I think. Rather than covering your face with makeup, people in Asia would much rather start with a clean and clear canvas. Therefore, prepping the skin was always important. The first product that I was introduced to was BB cream, which I think is a German invention for post-procedure skin. It was a skincare/makeup hybrid, which was then made popular by Korean beauty brands. I still remember my Skin79 BB creams! They only had one shade back then, but it did change my life, and introduced me to the world of K-beauty.

What is K-beauty for guys, and what are the most important aspects to know?

I think more conventionally, guys prefer a more subtle approach, good skin and full brows. For me, I emphasize skincare. My staples are always double cleansing and sunscreen in the daytime—always. Double cleansing really solved a lot of my skin issues.

It's when you use an oil-based cleanser to break down all that makeup and sunscreen, and then go in with another cleanser. You should do what's comfortable for you, though!

What are the essential products to kick-off your K-beauty journey?

I definitely think a good base starts off a K-beauty look. Moisturized skin and sunscreen is a must. I love using base products with skincare and sunscreen benefits. It's so innovative and convenient! Also any monochromatic blush and lip combos never go wrong.

Tell us about monolid eyes and how to enhance them.

I think traditionally people have always used terms like "open up" or "doelike" eyes to describe eyeshadow. These days, I don't really prescribe to those standards anymore. With more and more representation in the media, our monolids are finally having a moment to shine. I contour colors to elongate the eyelids even more. This is by taking a brush, taking eyeshadow, and extending your eye. You can use an eyeliner for this as well. Monolids are great for eyeshadow—it's a canvas that you can draw whatever you want on.

What are some tips when it comes to getting that signature dewy glow?

A hydrating toner and a sleeping mask at night do wonders! And if you can't do that, liquid highlighters that don't contain chunky glitters will do the trick. Mix them into your foundation or apply over with your fingers, but only on areas you want to accentuate. Too much can make you look . . . well, too much.

What are some tips you'd give when it comes to finding—discovering—your own signature look?

Experiment and play! Look for inspiration anywhere. Try different looks and see what makes you feel comfortable and confident.

K-POP: UNMASKING MASCULINITY

(1992-)

> *How Korean pop music allowed men everywhere to rethink makeup.*

WHEN BTS WON THE BILLBOARD MUSIC AWARD FOR TOP SOCIAL Artist in 2017, they did more than just crash the internet. Little did they know that they were waging a war against Western standards of masculinity.

The very next day, BTS was trending stateside, with thousands of Americans fixated by the guys' use of cosmetics and questioning their masculinity and sexualities.

While the Western world has been coming to grips with the gender binary under oppressive patriarchal rules more recently, South Korea has celebrated men and makeup on and off throughout history. Today, South Korean men purchase 20 percent of the world's beauty products. The country may be composed of only 25 million men, but collectively, they consume over a billion dollars' worth of cosmetics annually. On the streets from Seoul to Busan, it's normal to witness young men slathering their faces with cushion compact foundations, military guys buying sheet masks, or teens testing out red tints on their lips. For them, outward presentation and self-respect is the ultimate signifier of masculinity.

While South Korea may be a fine example of democratic beauty today, only three decades ago, wearing makeup as a man was considered taboo and was grounds for possible imprisonment for going against the country's strict Confucianism.

....

THE YEAR IS 1991, AND TWENTY-TWO-YEAR-OLD AMERICAN-born K-pop star Yang Joon-il, seeking the success he knew he wouldn't be able to achieve back in the US, performs onstage sporting an oversize printed jacket over a sleeveless black jumpsuit.

"My love, Rebecca," he croons, sweat dripping from his asymmetrical hair, down to his chin, eventually making its way to his bony clavicles. He slinks around the stage like a snake, rolling his body from side to side, his eyes hypnotic. He owns the stage, and watching his videos today, it's obvious that the seductive Yang is the epitome of a K-pop star.

But the audience, instead of roaring with applause, hisses, boos, and throws food at him. What gives?

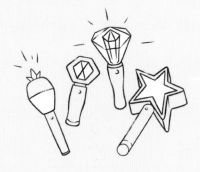

The country had spent the past three decades under the oppressive government of two authoritarian leaders, former presidents Park Chung Hee and Chun Doo-Hwan. Among Park's many suppressive acts, he had imprisoned men for growing their hair out too long. After Park was assassinated in 1980, Chun led a successful military coup and took control of the government. Protests against martial law and political suppression broke out in May, and in the city of Gwangju, Chun's violent crackdown on demonstrators, many of whom were students, resulted in the deaths of nearly 200 people (the exact number is disputed). Chun eventually lifted military control and became the country's president, though political suppression continued until 1988, when his term as president ended. One aspect that became popular was homegrown pop culture, a vehicle that helped provide moral support to many downtrodden South Korean youths. It didn't help Yang, whose unconventional look and Western style of music were still too far ahead of his time. Before he could even make a mark in music, South Korea turned its back on the singer, and he was forced to pack his bag and head back to the US, where he had immigrated at nine years old. His visa for reentry to Korea would be denied, and he settled in Florida, where he became a waiter. "I remember government officials telling me how embarrassed they were that I was Korean," he recalled later on a talk show.

While Yang may have been too flashy, only a year later a band called Seo Taiji and Boys would change the course of youth culture. The three-person band—composed of Seo, Yang Hyun-suk, and Lee Juno—introduced South Korea to a fusion of hip-hop, pop, new wave, and new jack swing beats. Soon enough, the band, with their baggy pants, gelled hair, and bad boy style, would be censored for being bad examples to young people. The group still became countercultural inspirations and icons of their era.

Four years later, a band called H.O.T. (High-Five of Teenagers) debuted, and surpassed Seo Taiji and Boys. They were handpicked by a producer named Lee Soo Man, who'd spent years studying youth culture and surveying young girls on what kind of idol they were looking for. Young people, disenchanted by the government and its stark, macho, militaristic portrayals of men, desired a gentler type of masculinity. As a result, the consensus was that their ideal heartthrob wasn't only handsome, wholesome, and innocent, but soft.

H.O.T. became a much-needed antidote to still hypermasculine Korean culture. Debuting with their saccharine first single, "Candy," the new bubblegum-pop sound with pretty-boy good looks, "cutesy" attitudes, and colorful outfits helped solidify them as South Korea's biggest pop culture icons ever.

The band would graduate to dyed locks and makeup for their second album, *Wolf and Sheep*. When they wore smoky eye makeup for their music video "I Yah!," it caused a governmental stir. Unnatural hair colors were banned from conservative networks like KBS (Korean Broadcasting System). But the look stuck around regardless, with more colorful boy bands to come, including Sechs Kies, g.o.d, Shinhwa, and Click-B. Soon enough, teenagers from all across the peninsula were inspired to test out their own looks, curious about the new beauty trends and eager to emulate them.

In 2003, a second, more international generation of K-pop groups began to take shape. Lee Soo Man was at it again, debuting a new five-member boy band called TVXQ! ("Rising Gods of the East!"). With TVXQ!, Lee ushered in a new era of *kkotminam,* aka "flower boys." (For more on the original flower boys, see page 43.) Kkotminam boys had delicate features, milky complexions, and dewy skin, and sang about innocent crushes. One of the lyrics from TVXQ!'s debut single, "Hug," was "Every day I want to be your cat." Whereas H.O.T. was pretty wholesome, these guys were veritable cherubs, with their permed hair, even-toned faces, and overall clean-cut style. This phase also ushered in other pretty boy groups like SS501, SHINee, Buzz, and Super Junior, among others, who would all use the same "flower boy" playbook.

But K-pop evolved quickly, and by the end of the 2000s, angelic-looking boys were no longer en vogue. They were soon eclipsed by the *jimseungdol,* aka "beast idols." These new K-pop groups had hard bodies, and would flaunt their washboard abs onstage. In a sea of beautiful flower boy types, jimseungdol stood out from the overcrowded pack. Bands like MBLAQ, Beast, and 2PM showcased more traditional masculinity, singing about seducing girls and making women fall in love with them, similar to the themes of Western pop songs.

But even so, makeup in Korean pop music continued to evolve as well. Despite their chiseled abs, most boy band members were rarely seen without smoky eyes, heavily drawn eyelids, and deep contouring. Their skin tones became sun-kissed and tanned, their hair shorter and shaggier. A breakout star from this era was Rain, a solo singer who became a sex symbol and was included in the TIME 100, *Time* magazine's list of the world's hundred most influential people, in 2011.

Behind the scenes, the South Korean government, realizing they had a cash cow on their hands, wanted in on the action. Once a critic of K-pop, the government started investing millions into the industry. By 2011, the government adopted K-pop under its Ministry of Culture, Sports and Tourism. Embassies and consulates throughout the world helped organize foreign K-pop concerts. K-pop stars became cultural ambassadors and the faces of the South Korean tourism industry.

South Korea took advantage of their growing soft power—with South Korea now "cool," in the eyes of the world, the government began sending out other industries on the K-pop wave. K-beauty would be pushed in tandem with K-pop's stars and their flawless complexions. (Think of BTS, which actively touts beauty products, and whose members are the face of many sheet mask, skincare, and cosmetics brands.) During the 2010s, boy bands would use makeup just as much as their female counterparts, and it became normal to witness guys with pastel-colored hair and shimmering, jewel-toned eyeshadows, lipstick, and blush on their faces. Bands like NCT 127, Pentagon, The Boyz, and TXT, among many others, all pushed the new era of male makeup forward. "There's no real difference between guys' and girls' makeup looks, except for maybe using less vibrant colors," says Yang Hui-yeon, the makeup artist for Pentagon. "Men are just as beautiful as women." Soon enough, South Korea dominated the beauty industry, once controlled by countries like France, the US, and Japan. Brands like AMOREPACIFIC and LG, as well as several indie brands, infiltrated the market—by the mid-2010s, K-beauty had arrived, with its sheet masks, essences, ampoules, snail mucin, and more.

With K-pop's dominance on the charts, preconceived notions of what men can and cannot be are being shattered. Today, K-pop has inspired people from around the world to partake in beautifying by painting their face, hair, and nails and becoming powerful in their own definition of sexy. Whether you're ready for it or not, prepare yourself for a continued beauty revolution.

HOW TO GET K-POP MAKEUP

A step-by-step guide.

Pentagon may be one of K-pop's newer boy bands, but the nine-member group is quickly becoming an internationally recognized act. The group, consisting of members Hui, Jinho, Hongseok, Shinwon, Yanan, Yeo One, Yuto, Kino, and Wooseok, has released bop-worthy singles including "Daisy," "Shine," and "Dr. Bebe." Their self-produced music is known for fusing hip-hop, pop, and trap flavors. Other than their music, the band has become known for their envelope-pushing beauty looks. In "Shine," it was high-intensity blush and freckles drawn in; "Dr. Bebe" showed a darker side of the band, with sexy, smoky eyes; and "Runaway" was all about rouged lips. About to hit the stage for your own K-pop performance? Read this how-to guide first. We got the lowdown on perfecting Pentagon's looks from the band's go-to makeup artist, Yang Hee-yeoun.

1. SKINCARE
Everything starts with skincare. For Yang, it's not about a 10-step regimen—more like three (see page 48 for more on the Korean 10-step regimen). "I'll start with toner, moisturizer, and a water-based cream and put as much needed," she says. "For dryer skin, I'll apply some essence."

2. PRIMER
Before applying any makeup, Yang will use a face primer. "After skincare, the trick is using a good primer that absorbs any of the skin's extra oil." A good primer will also create a solid base, Yang says, "so that nothing cracks or creases."

3. FOUNDATION
It might seem counterintuitive, but the secret behind foundation is not applying too much. Instead, it's about finding thick, waterproof, long-wearing formulas. "Again, because idols sweat so much, we'll want a foundation that can withstand the elements onstage," says Yang. The K-pop way to apply? Use a brush.

4. CONTOURING
Koreans call this "shading," but the concept is the same. It's all about making a more chiseled face. "Idols' faces can look bigger under stage lights, so I'll outline areas that need a little more shading," Yang says. "I'll put the face under a light, and emphasize the areas that hit the shadows." For K-pop stars, it's mostly about elongating the nose and creating a more chiseled jaw.

5. EYES
Depending on the concept and look, Yang will either use eyeliner or just eyeshadow. For eyeliner, the look is to lightly draw the lower lids. Then it's about using eyeshadow to elongate the eye outward. Warmer tones are popular for K-pop stars—think copper, reds, burnt oranges, and browns. Try going with the lightest color first and then blend in darker shades.

6. LIPS
For K-pop stars, the juicier lips, the sexier the look. Yang says she'll use a lip tint rather than a lipstick so that it lasts longer. She'll start in the middle of the lips and blend outward. Generally it's a pink or subtle red shade. For Pentagon's "Runaway" video, it was deep reds. "But it's all about the concept we're going for," she says. And remember: the stage is different from photoshoots or editorials. For the latter, opt for softer lipsticks—they'll look more natural in photos.

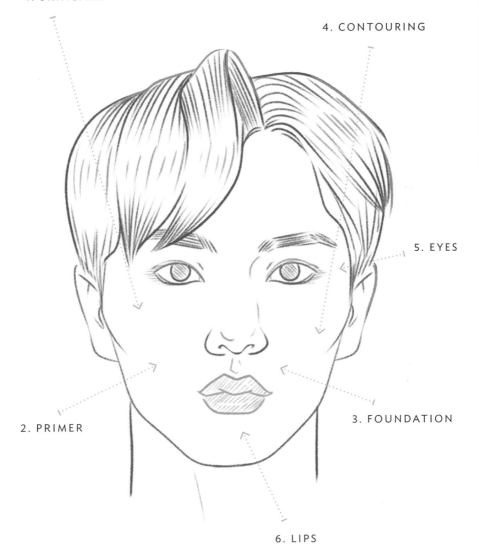

1. SKINCARE

4. CONTOURING

5. EYES

3. FOUNDATION

2. PRIMER

6. LIPS

FIVE MINUTES WITH HOLLAND, K-POP'S FIRST OPENLY GAY IDOL

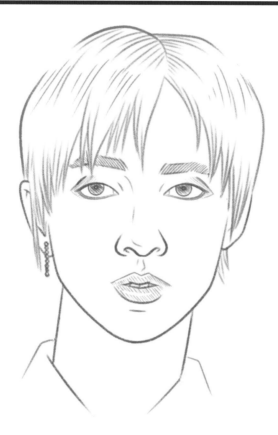

Holland made waves when he debuted as the first openly gay K-pop idol in South Korea. His music video "Neverland," hit airwaves in 2018 with full montages of him making out with another man, tongue and all—this was historic. While it may not be big news stateside, for South Korea, a relatively conservative country where LGBTQIA rights are limited, this was shocking. Quickly, the video was taken off television stations and given the "19+" adult rating.

Though there are gay K-pop stars, none have been open about their sexualities. So for Holland to not only come out *before* his debut, but to be forthright about who he was and has always been, signaled that a cultural shift is brewing in South Korea.

Today, Holland is still one of the only openly gay K-pop idols. While we hope for a day when simply *being* isn't an act of bravery, we commend Holland for being a pioneer and putting his life and career on the line to pursue freedom. We spoke to Holland about gender roles, his views of masculinity, and, of course, makeup!

You're inspiring a new generation of young people to become more comfortable in their own skin. How did you come to owning both your masculinity and your femininity?

In Korea, the notion of self-care and beauty care is regarded as an obvious and natural concept by all genders. Through self-care, one can naturally find and come into their own sense of style that matches them. I think that's why a lot of Koreans pursue natural makeup, the "softest" things that best suit us. It's less about masculinity and more about what will best suit us in a natural way.

If you closely analyze the process of self-care for all genders, in everything from styling hair and trimming nails to perfume selection, it is ultimately a way through which each person's unique flair and color seeps through. Makeup, then, is not just for women or necessarily feminine.

Tell us about beauty and how it relates to your freedom of expression. What makeup products do you use in real life, onstage, or in your photos/videos?

I regard makeup as one avenue of self-expression. I think true beauty is when my confidence in self-expression is able to show through visually. Everyone has a best version of themselves that they want to achieve. Makeup is an avenue through which we can fulfill our preferences and maximize our strongest features. In my daily life, I frequently use MAC Cosmetics: the bold colors, the lasting coverage, and color development are all very nice. It helps me to better express myself. I also really like Boy de Chanel's foundation base.

How do you think K-pop has positively pushed men to become more comfortable with their beauty?

In addition to dance and music, both beauty and other visual elements achieved through makeup and fashion are crucial components in the K-pop business as well. I think makeup is a medium through which we are able to add more color and perfect art. Should I call this the "coloring" process? Makeup is not only helping artists' in the music industry better establish their identities, but it's also playing an important role in the movie industry, and pretty much in everything that requires a visual element. Total beauty is achieved by having both inner and outer beauty. So it's difficult to define the exact meaning, but the more beautiful something is, the greater the impression it makes, right?

Korea is a country with rapid economic and cultural development. We were able to cultivate and refine our aesthetic eye, and we put a lot of effort into detecting and getting ahead of cultural trends. So maybe that's why K-pop, the center of the Korean wave, has been reinventing art in a new way, through visual convergence since the 1990s when the K-pop group H.O.T. set a unique precedent with their futuristic makeup concepts and unusual hairstyling.

Finally, how is makeup changing culture for the better?

You can achieve the image or look that you desire while also respecting and admiring the preferences and individuality of others—makeup that touches on art can open your eyes to a variety of colors. Just hearing someone tell you "You look beautiful" has the power to make us so happy.

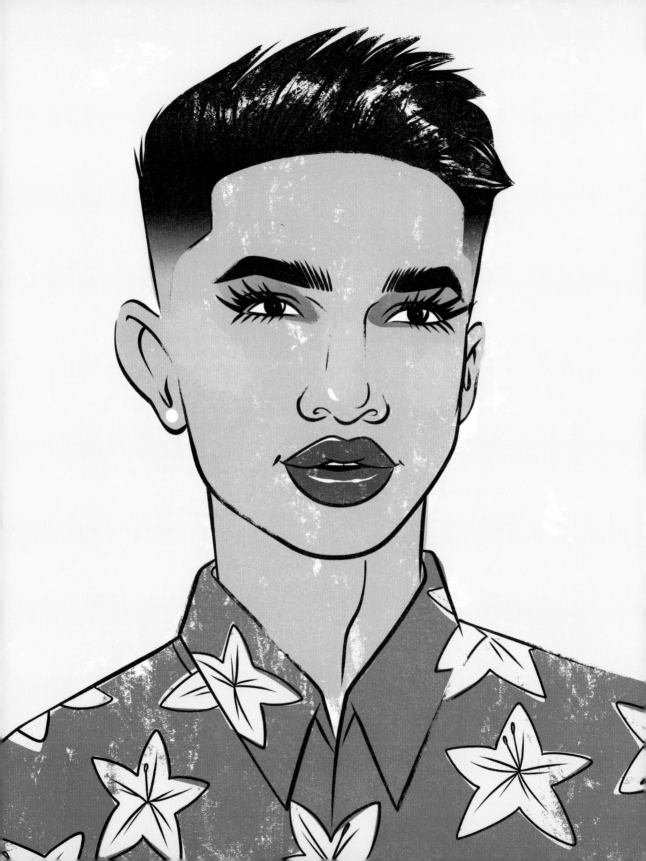

BRETMAN ROCK

(1 9 9 8 -)

How a Hawaiian tween became the most beloved beauty guru.

LOS ANGELES IS BETTER KNOWN AS *GLOSS ANGELES*—THE sticky, addictive, bubblegum-pink beauty mecca of the entire world. Thousands of miles away on the breezy island of O'ahu lives one of the biggest names in beauty, the Filipinx American influencer Bretman "Da Baddest" Rock.

For Bretman, maintaining a semblance of normalcy is completely necessary for survival. Not only for his mental health, but for the sake of others. "I feel like if I moved to LA I would be on every tea channel every day because I'm so outspoken and I'm just like, if you wanna fight, bitch, we will be fighting," he says with a smile. "So I'm kinda doing everyone a favor by staying home."

And home has always been Hawaii, where he's surrounded by his childhood friends and his family. "They're the ones who tell me how unfunny I am and keep it real," he says. As the story goes, Bretman gained instant fame in the eighth grade when the first video he posted on YouTube went viral. The video showcases a fearlessly *real* tween popping off on his camera, just talking about life. "I had 10,000 followers then and thought I was seriously famous," he recalls. "I'm like, 'teacher, don't you know I have 10,000 followers, I really have to turn this in?'" From there, his social media presence exploded, and almost overnight, he was flying around the world. The Philippines one day, New York City the next, endorsing beauty products, shelling out #sponsored content, making appearances, and securing the bag—this, all before he was even legal to vote.

Since then, he's been named the People's Choice "Beauty Influencer of 2019," sealed partnerships with brands like Wet n Wild, and filmed an MTV show about his life. The young star's proven that he's one of Gen Z's most influential and fearless voices. In the following interview with Bretman, we talk shop, delve into beauty—and even shed a few tears along the way. The conversation reveals that behind his beat face, those false eyelashes, and that devilish smile is a young man who just wants to be *seen*.

Bretman, it's so good to finally sit down with you. Tell me about your come-up story.

Ugh, I don't even know. I feel so old nowadays. There's like new influencers coming out every day, which I fucking love, honestly. It's so cool to see more boys in beauty because when I was starting off, I was really one of the only men that I knew in makeup.

When did you first wear makeup?

Shoutout to my grandma, the one person that is still my day one. I would always watch her getting ready for church. I would literally just sit on her bed watching her put on makeup. We lived in the Philippines then, but I still remember even if I close my eyes. I can still see her putting on the three lipsticks that she had, layering them, and the blushes that she had. She put blush on me and I felt so fishy going to church.

Grandma inspired everything—how did your parents come around?

My family always, always, always, *always* knew I was gay. When I turned four my mom and my dad bought me this toy truck that I could drive. Inside the trunk were Barbies. I realize it now, but my parents always knew I was gay.

When you were a kid, you must have been fearless.

I have always just been in front of the camera. Whenever I'm in front of the camera I've always been Bretman Fucking Rock. I've always made videos. I was in eighth grade when I posted my very first video ever on YouTube. I thought I was a fucking fashion icon. I would post lookbooks, "Bretman's spring/summer lookbook," as if we had fall and winter in Hawaii. After, I'd always ask everyone on Facebook if they could share it. My mom would tell all her coworkers that her son's a YouTuber with thirty subscribers.

That confidence must have been so impressive, now that you think about it.

If I'm being honest, there are days when I am jealous of my younger self. Before social media, I only had my other peers, and they were always so encouraging. I was so confident as a kid. And now, I just feel like ever since I've been on social media, people will ruin you sometimes, and as confident as I like to portray myself, I just think that I gave less fucks when I was younger. I just felt so much more normal, if that makes sense.

I wouldn't say that I'm not confident anymore. I would say like my younger self was so much more free, and I have videos of me late to school and [with a] full face of makeup. I really thought I was the fiercest bitch in school.

Tell me about cancel culture. Have you ever felt canceled? Have people ever come after you?

Yes. That's kind of a hard question. Last week, an old video of mine resurfaced. I said the N-word five years ago in videos. I'm not even gonna try and sugarcoat it—videos, with an "s." And this was before cancel culture was even a thing. I got approached by this woman and she's like, you're so bright but you need to stop saying this word—it's not your word, it's not for you. At the time, even though I wasn't really educated on what she was saying, I felt what she was saying and I knew that I fucked up. I knew what I did was wrong. This was even before someone saw these videos. I'm not trying to make up excuses, but some of those songs and videos were of me rapping to songs or me re-creating [music] videos. Like I already said, I apologized about it so many times. It's ignorant then as it is ignorant now. I've grown from that, and if you guys wanna cancel me, cancel the fifteen-year-old Bretman Rock, not the twenty-one-year-old Bretman Rock, because he's not that Bretman Rock anymore. He doesn't even have those gap teeth anymore, he doesn't even have that acne anymore, and he can color match his foundation now.

I've apologized about it the minute that I posted it. I've apologized every year after that. Because I was ignorant, a part of me is still ignorant. I feel like I'm still slowly and always growing. I feel like cancel culture doesn't give you the opportunity to grow. Because once you say something or once you do something bad, they'll attack you and beat you down until you don't even want to do what you do anymore.

How are you dealing with mental health while being so visible on social media?

I don't even know if I'm doing that, if I'm being honest with you. Negative comments and the whole cancel culture thing—it's a big deal. Social media is affecting a lot of people's mental health, and I will say it has kinda affected me more than I thought it would. I just try not to share so much anymore. I really genuinely only try to share the light in my life. I don't really like to show too much, just because I feel like you get what you put out. I feel if I put out great energy, I will get that back, and obviously if I'm a negative person online and if I'm always complaining about everything, that just comes back to me, honestly.

What would you say to someone who doesn't know who you are, and how would you introduce yourself?

I would say, "Hi, I'm Bretman Rock, I'm just a Leo and I think that's all you need to know about me."

Skincare or makeup?

Skincare, girl. As much as I love makeup, skincare is where it's at. Because if you really want your makeup to come through, your skin gotta be popping. You must have a cute base to have a cute face. Period.

Best skincare tip you have?

Three fucking letters, bitch: S.P.F. At *least* 50, especially if you're a Hawaiian girl.

First crush?

First gay crush was Jafar from *Aladdin* and his big, big bird. And my first straight crush would have to be Kim Possible. If we're talking real people, my first girl crush would be Mila Kunis, and my first guy crush would be the Rock. I was actually named after the Rock.

What sparks joy?

Right now, my plants, my boyfriend, and food.

Pizza or *pancit*?

Girl. Next question. You already know the fucking answer.

Favorite app on your phone?

Right now I have been obsessed with the app called Picture This. You take a picture of any plant and it identifies the plant for you. It tells you how to take care of it and stuff like that. But if it has to do with social media I would say Instagram and TikTok.

Tea or coffee?

Coffee, but I love spilling the tea.

Face masks or sheet masks?

Face masks. Sheet masks are too cold sometimes, and it slips off, you know what I mean? Have you ever had like a face mask kinda come down, and you're like, okay, bitch.

Guilty pleasure?

I would say doing my makeup. Whenever I'm feeling sad, sometimes there's days I do my makeup three times because I want to practice. Whenever I'm having a bad day I just do my makeup.

While we've been conditioned to wear sunscreen in the summer to places like the beach or the pool, it's a common misconception that you only need it when it's sunny out—you actually need it all year-round. (Think about it: the sun is beaming even in the cold winter months.) The sun's UVA and UVB rays are toxic, and too much exposure can cause skin cancer at worst, and aging, sunburn, and hyperpigmentation at best. Here's everything you needed to know about SPF—and more.

WHAT'S IN A NAME?

SPF stands for "sun protection factor," and the number that follows it represents how much longer it protects your skin from damage vs. the length of time it takes for your unprotected skin to get burned. For instance, if you usually get some kind of burn after 10 minutes in the sun, you can multiply that by the SPF number to estimate how long you can be in the sun after applying sunscreen before burning (or ideally, before reapplying your sunscreen). If it's an SPF 30 in this example, it would be 10 x 30 = 300 minutes of protection. Of course, this isn't a foolproof formula for everyone, and doesn't take into account the long-term effects of sun exposure. That's because the sun emits two types of UV radiation: ultraviolet A (UVA) and ultraviolet B (UVB). Though they damage skin in different ways, both are toxic and can lead to cancer. UVB has a shorter wavelength that penetrates only the top layer of your skin, the epidermis, which is how it causes burning. UVA has a longer wavelength—it penetrates through to the second layer of your skin, the dermis, and is therefore most associated with skin aging, but doesn't cause sunburn. That means the SPF number on your sunscreen isn't relevant to UVA exposure, so to prevent sun damage, you'll want to find a sunscreen with "broad spectrum" on the label, meaning it gives you protection against both UVA and UVB radiation. When using SPF, numbers really do matter—though, anything above SPF 50 really is just marketing. AKA you don't need anything above SPF 50. Just look at this graph:

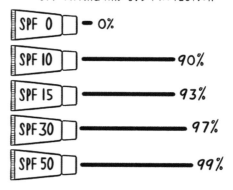

SPF RATING AND UVB PROTECTION

SPF 0 — 0%
SPF 10 — 90%
SPF 15 — 93%
SPF 30 — 97%
SPF 50 — 99%

TWO TYPES OF SUNSCREEN

You may have read that sunscreen comes in two types: chemical and physical. You can think of chemical sunscreens like a sponge that absorbs the sun's rays, while physical sunscreens act more like an umbrella to deflect radiation from the skin. Which is best for you? Depends on what you're looking for.

The general consensus is that physical sunscreen is less harsh and won't cause inflammation if you have acne-prone or sensitive skin. But it's also thicker, and the ingredients—zinc oxide and/or titanium oxide—can leave that dreaded gray cast on your skin and sometimes make your skin feel sticky. Physical sunscreen also needs to be reapplied more often, as it isn't sweatproof, although it's effective immediately after application. Chemical sunscreen doesn't leave behind any residue and usually blends in seamlessly. But its active ingredients—oxybenzone, avobenzone, octisalate, homosalate, octocrylene, octinoxate—can cause skin irritation, in addition to clogging pores. Some of the most popular ingredients in chemical sunscreens have also been found to be toxic to the environment and possibly the body. And keep in mind that chemical sunscreen takes 20 minutes to be effective post-application.

There's been a recent debate within the skincare industry around chemical sunscreens: not only can they irritate skin, but they can also damage the environment. For instance, studies have shown that oxybenzone and octinoxate, common ingredients in chemical sunscreens, contribute to the depletion of coral reefs. Many are now pushing toward safer ingredients like zinc oxide and titanium dioxide, both found in physical sunscreens.

BEST PRACTICES?

Apply and reapply often. Studies have shown that even with SPF 100, sunburn can occur. When applying, use an ample amount—for your face, that's a lima bean–size dollop. If you're wearing makeup, apply sunscreen first as your base, and layer all other products on top. Try to apply 15 minutes before you plan to head outside. Note that wearing sunscreen alone without a hat or clothing, means you're still never completely safe from the harmful effects of the sun, but reapplying sunscreen throughout the day, every two hours or immediately after sweating or exposure to water, will help keep your skin safe.

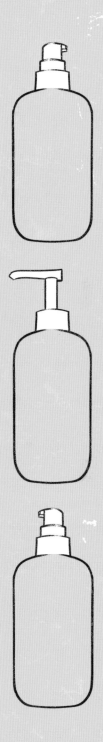

WHAT I LOVE ABOUT ME

Ten Pretty Boys on how they came to self-acceptance and love.

Now that we've gone through history and back to uncover pretty boys far and wide, we invite you to meet a few *real-life* examples: the pretty boys next door.

As you've read in this book, being a pretty boy is so much more than your physical appearance or the cosmetics you may use to express yourself—it's not so easily defined. Rather, it's about embracing *you* for *you,* fully understanding your entire, vibrant, authentic self from the inside out. We hope these unique stories will inspire you on your own journey of self-love and discovery, and toward understanding your masculinity on your own terms.

1. *Isaiah Piche*,

Whittier, California, *writer*

....

I AM DISABLED AND GAY—AND I LOVE EVERY BIT OF MYSELF. However, coming to terms with my identities, and loving myself for them, is a continuous journey. There is something to be said about being gay and disabled in a patriarchal society—that is, a society dominated by able-bodied white men.

I have cerebral palsy. My disability is the result of negligent professional care during my birth. I was left drowning in my mother's womb while doctors insisted on a natural delivery. Consequently, we were rushed into a C-section, but it was too late. The damage was done.

I identify as a "man" with intent. I identify as a man because society says disabled men are not really "men." I identify as a man because society says gay men should be persecuted. I identify as a man because I am a first-generation Latinx American, and my father is a man, and my grandfather was a wonderful man. I identify as a man because society says disabled gay Latino men do not exist. I identify as a man because I am a man.

My families are immigrants from Mexico and El Salvador. Therefore, like many other cultures, Latinx culture reproduces gender inequality due to patriarchy. In other words, "boys" and "girls" are brought up accordingly. My earliest memory of going against this norm involves me playing with my mother's and grandmother's high heels. I would hobble around the house and entertain myself with four-inch stilettos. I could not play like this around the men in my family, however. I was frowned upon when I was caught.

Today I've come to love myself. I know I look good. I am beautiful. I am a disabled gay king. Part of me trying to stay healthy is by repeating affirmations. I think of things to be grateful for, pray and meditate in the morning. I also exercise daily. I have realized that maintaining my peace is crucial, and it's a huge part of maintaining self-love. I know that being a "pretty boy," that being a man, allows me to help spread the message.

2. *Christopher Hadley*,

New York City, *student*

THE EARLIEST MEMORY I HAVE OF BEING TRANS ISN'T EVEN MY own. When I came out to my best friend, she reminded me that I would ask her whenever we stayed up late to talk, if she would still be my friend if I were a boy.

I couldn't make up a better origin story if I tried. Back then, though, I was terrified to ask this question. I would tell her (in a much less elegant way, because I was maybe eight), "I would still be me. Like my personality, all of the same memories, but I was a boy." She's still my best friend, so I guess the answer was yes.

I have a tumultuous relationship with my own transness. As many do, I find myself falling into my internalized transphobia much more often than I'd like to admit. I once told a friend that I didn't understand trans Pride, because it wasn't like it was a good thing to be trans—it just meant you were born wrong. As I grow up, I'm constantly trying to unlearn those internal transphobic instincts.

Even living in New York City, there have been cruel moments with strangers just on the street. One of my best friends is a girl called Frances. She came to visit me on Valentine's Day at my school in Bay Ridge. It's about a 45-minute train ride from Jay Street–MetroTech, which is the stop by her school. She brought me flowers, I brought her a book of poetry. Our joke is that everyone in the world thinks we're dating. On the train ride back together, on our way to Fortune House for dumplings, a woman across from us beckoned for my attention. I looked at her and she asked me, "Are you guys lesbians?" It was a punch in the gut. I shook my head, but I knew I had turned bright red, I knew I didn't look convincing. She asked instead, "Oh, so you guys aren't together? But you *are* lesbians, right?"

I checked out a little after that. I know I told her, "No. I'm a dude." (I use "dude" sometimes because it feels nonthreatening. Also, because I feel weird calling myself a "man" when I look like I'm fourteen on a good day. I'm working on it.) And I know that after that, she began listing all the reasons I couldn't be a man. A punch list of my biggest insecurities, both about my actual corporeal being and the way that I carried myself.

Today, as for defining my own masculinity—it's been a necessity from the start. I was never going to be the same boy that my brother is: sporty, charismatic, etc. So in some regards, that's felt like less of a challenge. My real mission is to be the type of man that I am proud of. Someone like my dad, who is gentle and intense in the way that he loves people, who is empathetic and strong.

3. *Micah Cyrus*,

Los Angeles, *television writer*

....

GROWING UP, I HAD A SKEWED IDEA ABOUT BEING TRADITION-ally masculine. Both my dad and brother were alpha males who served as role models for the interests and behaviors that I should adapt. The underlying problem was that I wasn't interested in the things they were passionate about: sports, the outdoors, chasing women. It was hard for me to grasp my place in the world, especially when I sought their validation and approval and didn't find it until much later in life.

I began to tell myself and others that I wanted to live the life my heart believes it should. If that means wearing concealer or wearing nail polish—I choose to follow my heart's desires. My understanding of Black masculinity growing up was rooted in the understanding that I must walk with my chest high, not be vulnerable, and feed into the idea that homophobia was socially acceptable. I no longer subscribe to any of that. Today, Black masculinity is unique to who you are as a Black man, if that's walking in stilettos or with your chest out, not being afraid to tell someone how you *really* feel, or loving our brothers for whoever they might be sexually attracted to. I'd like to tell others the same thing I wish I told myself growing up: whenever someone tells you that your truth is abnormal, understand they are only operating with a narrow lens rooted in ignorance or hate. Help them find love by being true to yourself. I want to take self-love to a chapter of my life that isn't afraid of the barriers that come with romantic relationships. The second that I started telling myself that I'm a beautiful Black man was the first step toward being truly vulnerable romantically. I know my person will serve as a positive reinforcement to the man I can now confidently look in the mirror and love.

4. *Kemio Kurosawa,*

Tokyo, *model and influencer*

MY PARENTS PASSED AWAY WHEN I WAS TWO AND I NEVER GOT to know them. And so I was raised by my grandparents in Tokyo. Growing up I always knew I was different in many ways. For one, I didn't look Japanese. My hair was always curly and my features weren't so typically Japanese. I only discovered I was Italian and Persian as well and the details of my parents when I was in high school. My mother was full Japanese, but my father was from Italy and Iran. [My grandparents] only kept these details from me because being half in Japan during childhood is tough. [My grandmother] didn't want to hurt me by telling me I may be different.

But it's being different that allowed me to thrive. I started recording Vine videos when that was still a thing, and comedy became my calling. Soon enough, I became a viral star and then moved on to television. Though I gained so many followers and people started recognizing me as a celebrity, I wanted to experience much more. At twenty, I decided to move to Los Angeles, a place where I felt in my fantasies was where I could be free. I launched a YouTube channel and it took off. It was in LA that I felt I could really be authentically myself. Seeing as so many of my friends were free, I thought that I would have the courage as well. And so I came out only to my close friends.

After a year in LA, I went home and came out to my grandparents. At first, they didn't like it. My point in telling them wasn't to hurt them; rather, to share with them my truth. I later released my first book in Japan, where I came out as gay to Japan. When it hit shelves it really surprised me. I didn't know that it would be such a big deal. It became national news. There were so many articles of "Kemio coming out as gay." Japan is still a relatively straight culture, and so for someone in the public eye to be [out as] gay is still a big deal.

In retrospect, I realize that coming out is different to every person. I do want to say there's no rush for anyone to do so. You don't need to come out. And if you do, do it for yourself, knowing that you're no different for being gay and that there isn't anything wrong with being gay. I was so scared before I came out, but afterward felt so much support. Just know that there is another side and the consequences are good and happy. It does get better.

5. *Jasjyot Singh Hans,*

Delhi, India, *illustrator*

....

I'VE ALWAYS THOUGHT I WAS UNDESIRABLE. I WAS ALWAYS FAT, and fat people don't have very many multidimensional portrayals in the media. They're either there to be the butt of a joke or a sidekick. That contributed to the way I felt about myself growing up, like I wasn't of value. As I grew into a boy who liked boys, I felt like an alien with no one to talk to. I got bullied in school, and was made to feel like nothing.

I'm also Sikh, and proudly wear a turban because it connects me to my history, who I am, and where I come from. I also get to wear them in any darn color I want and look fabulous! Post-9/11 in the US, the turban has been seen as a symbol of violence and hate, but that speaks to people's ignorance of things and people outside their country, because the Sikh religion is about equality, peace, and love. Most people think Sikhs are Muslims. I have faced hate and racism, but I am quick to brush it off. I'm happy to speak about my turban, my people, and my Sikh identity to people if I feel they're willing to listen and learn. But a lot of times people are so hostile that they don't want to know more and stay ignorant. That is a mindset in which there's no space for learning and understanding.

Today, I'm continuing to practice self-love but working hard at it and staying true to myself. I have always had a complicated relationship with the word "ugly" and the way it is used to marginalize physical traits in communities, tribes, and races. To me, true ugliness is in the mind of the speaker, not the recipient, in those conversations. What has conventionally been taught to us as ugly is often the very thing that is beautiful. I can proudly say today that yes, I am worthy.

6. *Ady Del Valle,*

Boston, *Big and Tall model*

I'VE BEEN REJECTED AND TOLD MANY THINGS BY MANY PEOPLE throughout my life, even in the industry, because of my size. Feeling unworthy or even unattractive took a long toll on me. I was depressed and in a dark space in my life in my teens and early twenties. I would not want to go out with friends or hang out, and I felt like I was a bother or would ruin plans because I felt less than. I was so insecure with my large chest, my stomach, the pigmentation in certain parts of my body.

As I was battling my self-worth, I was also confronting my sexuality in being a gay man and feeling like I couldn't come out. I was scared my family wouldn't want me or I'd be rejected by friends.

I was around twenty-eight when I had a moment one day and said to myself, "I can't do this anymore. I have to live for me while I'm still young." I pursued doing things I love, and that's when I found the Ady I wanted to be. Modeling has helped me become my own person and what I want to be in the world. I feel beautiful when I do what I love most, because I can help others that look like me feel the same. I defined my own beauty by just being me and doing what I've imagined in real life.

Today, beauty to me has no meaning; beauty is in the eye of the beholder. And all of me is beautiful—my large chest, my stomach, my gay identity—I am so proud of it all.

7. *Innanoshe Richard Akuson,*

Kwanga, Nigeria, *advocate*

I LIKE TO THINK THAT I'M A GLORIOUS MANIFESTATION OF MY name, Innanoshe, which means "a gift from God" in my native Koro language.

When I think about growing up in Nigeria, there's this cloud of ambivalence that shrouds my memories, which I struggle to articulate. Some days I remember my childhood with great fondness; other days, I profoundly regret it. My father, I imagine, attempted to "toughen" me out of love, knowing full well the world that awaited me outside the comfort of the life he and my mother afforded us. In school, people poked fun at me. In university, after a close friend outed me, I became a social pariah—the poster child of "homos." That incident infantilized me in a way that rendered me as helpless as I was back in primary and boarding school.

I think having to move to America for safety after surviving a homophobic incident in Nigeria brought me to my knees. I was forced to leave the careful life that I'd created for myself, the friends I'd come to know and love, and, more importantly, my family. But the move has also changed me in many ways that I'm the better for.

Interestingly, I never considered myself inherently ugly; I always believed my beauty or people's perception of it, or lack thereof, was contextual. I had a strongly held belief that in a different space and amongst different people, I would be seen as objectively beautiful. So, I nurtured that belief carefully and closely to my heart as I went through puberty, adolescence, and acne for years. The older I got, and the more I discovered my smarts and wit, I became less occupied with my physical appearance.

In America, I've seen the radiance and beauty I always knew I possessed affirmed not only by others, but also by myself. Every day I look into the mirror, I'm reminded of the rocky emotional and mental journey that brought me this point, where I can stare at my reflection and enjoy every bit of it.

At this point in my life and based on my personal experience, I'd say beauty is a total alignment of a person's inward and outward radiance; a result of which is a cooling and peaceful self-assuredness that has quieted the waters of my soul. It's honestly whatever you want it to be. Today, I'm allowing the hard-won kindness and love I feel for myself to lead the way. I refuse to preempt or dictate anything.

8. MRSHLL Marshall Bang,

Seoul, South Korea, *Singer*

....

I'M FROM CALIFORNIA AND HAD SOMEHOW GOTTEN A CHANCE to become a singer in Korea. I came out to the world in a big magazine in Korea in 2015.

This was a big deal. As a new singer, it was considered risky, especially in a country where being outwardly queer is still unacceptable. There also wasn't a precedent for it. No one in the Korean music industry had come out before.

It was important to me because I didn't want gossip or tabloid fodder deterring the public away from me as an artist. Not only that, my parents are both super religious—my mother is an ordained minister.

On a personal level, I didn't want to hide any more. I wanted to start dating. I didn't want my mom to find out from other channels like someone saying to her, "Pastor, do you know your son was seen with another guy?"

When the magazine finally published it wasn't only big news in South Korea—it was huge news back home in California. My parents were upset. My mom freaked out and she sent me these sad messages that broke me. But they also started a conversation between us. I attended a Christian university so I'm pretty well-versed about biblical stuff and scripture. She went to a rival private Christian university and has her own beliefs. After many debates, we came to a stalemate situation where neither side was willing to budge. We couldn't discredit each other because we knew what the hell we were talking about.

Though they're not the most accepting, my parents still support and love me the best way they know how. I realized now that I'm a little older, I don't necessarily need their approval. I'm self-sufficient and confident in who I am and have my chosen family to support me.

I also have my fans. This is why visibility is so important anywhere. I get messages everyday with queer folx in Korea DMing me how they're empowered just by seeing someone like me. I do see it as important that there are people like me and Holland to be out there doing our thing.

I'm loud and proud but know that not everyone is in my position. For those out there coming into their own, know that nothing happens overnight. We're all growing as human beings and trying to figure out how we fit into this tapestry of life. Also, don't feel you need to live in shame to live your life. You are powerful how you are.

9. *Mohammed Attiyeh,*

New Jersey, *graduate student*

....

I WAS FIVE YEARS OLD WHEN 9/11 HAPPENED. IT WAS NOT until I was in high school that I faced my first racist attack. A fellow student referred to me and my family as terrorists. At first, it did not bother me, until I realized that he truly believed what he was saying. Luckily, my football teammates were next me when this scene occurred, and they came to my defense—they also debunked any stereotypes or misconception that student had against Muslims.

It's nothing new. The men in my family were called every racist slur toward Muslim Arabs that you can think of—these included terrorist, camel jockey—while also being victims of police brutality. The women in my family were discriminated [against] at their places of work because they were wearing hijabs and it was clear they were Muslim.

I have been discriminated [against] in courts as a young Arab Muslim and received harsher penalties and fines compared to young white men who received a ticket for the same offenses. I once walked into a restaurant in Boston and was never served as every white person in there continued to stare and whisper at my cousins and me. I have been in several fights that resulted from racism where an older white male looked at my cousin and said, "Who do you think you are talking to? Do you see the color of my skin?!"

The darkest moment in my life was when I became a father at the age of nineteen. It was with a girl I was supposed to get engaged to and was dating at the time. Of course, my family found out and they were beyond disappointed. To them, I messed up every "Muslim rule" possible, and they thought I was going to be a failure. And for a while I believed them. I became depressed after my family couldn't bear to look at me and at how I "ruined my entire life" by getting a girl pregnant.

I fell into depression and also almost failed a semester of school at the time, and couldn't hold a job. I sought counseling, something not common in Muslim culture, where there is so much stigma around mental illness. To the older generations, if you had a mental illness, that meant that you weren't "close to God."

After counseling, the phrases that stuck in my head were "Everything happens for a reason" and "Everything is going to be okay." It was repeating those phrases to myself that I realized I have to work extremely hard to find my self-worth. One day soon I hope to consider myself beautiful, but until then, will continue working on myself.

10. *Edgar Fabian Frias,*

Tulsa, Oklahoma, *healer*

....

GROWING UP, I ALWAYS FELT DIFFERENT AND THIS DIFFERENCE often made me feel alienated, ugly, and unseen. As a baby, I was born with a bad case of rheumatic fever and with congenital strabismus. Doctors feared that I would not survive or that I would be left with developmental challenges in my life. Thankfully, I did survive but grew up knowing that my appearance often made me stand out. My parents, both undocumented immigrants from Mexico, never had the money to help me have surgery for my strabismus, so I grew up with my eyes appearing different than others. Doctors marveled at my ability to detect depth in spaces even though my eyes were not able to do it physically. "Your brain is filling in all the details," some doctors would say to me.

Despite the deep love and care I received from my parents, I often felt incredibly ugly as a child. I resonated so profoundly with the story of the ugly duckling and wished so hard that I would also have the same type of outcome as them. This story gave me so much hope at a time when I felt utterly powerless and unloved. On top of that, I was tall for my age, fat, brown, and was interested in so many non-normative things and always felt expansive in my gender, although I did not have the language for that at a young age.

Thankfully, I have had the privilege and honor of receiving so much healing in my life, through the love of friends, my queer, transgender, nonbinary, and gender expansive communities, therapy, ceremony, and through the grace of Goddexx.

I have been able to embrace my difference with joy. I am a nonbinary brujx, a child of indigenous (Wixárika) healers and medicine people, a joyous creatrix, a smuggler of information and concepts across time, space, and cognitive regimentations. The mutant magick I share with others through my contemporary art practice; my online spells; my work as an educator, psychotherapist, and curator; and through the other avenues I traverse is forging new dimensions in collaboration with others. My life's praxis has created a world where my visions, dreams, and entire being are celebrated and cherished.

Today, I am no longer unseen. I am seen. I am no longer ugly. I am prismatic. I have become the beautiful swan I used to yearn to be as a child. I am proof that the things you have been shamed for are your greatest gifts and that the things you were made to fear and hate about yourself are the very things that others will adore and cherish about you.

Acknowledgments

By the time this is written, published, and shipped, Good Light beauty will have been birthed into the world. It's a beauty brand for Pretty Boys—and those from all identities—to celebrate who they are and shine in their own *good light*.

It's humbling to think how my business has expanded in the past four years. When I launched Very Good Light in October 2016, I hadn't a clue that it would resonate with so many people. There was so much pushback in those early days with naysayers commenting how this idea would never work. But like so many hard-headed entrepreneurs, I threw caution to the wind and trekked forth into the unknown, sustained on hope and the kindness of friends who cheered me along—although I'm sure, they, too, were uncertain of my life choice.

This journey hasn't been easy. In the early days, I sublet my Brooklyn apartment, sold some of my vintage clothing, scrounged up the $7,000 in my bank account and put it all towards launching the site. In weeks I became homeless, relying on friends who lent me their couches and provided me with home-cooked meals. In those early days, I lugged my entire life around New York City in two heavy suitcases, hustling uptown and downtown, taking meetings to get Very Good Light off the ground. But still, I kept my struggle close to my chest, as if it was a shameful secret that needed to be layered in lavish silks so no one would know the emptiness underneath. No one knew how much I doubted myself—not my sister, my parents, or those who followed my "glamorous" life on Instagram.

Those early days took grit, but more so: passion. In retrospect I could only have done this in my twenties—risk-taking later in life is just too exhausting. But what sustained me was this small but quickly growing community that Very Good Light cultivated. Week by week it only grew. Our first month had 30,000 visitors, but by month three we had 100,000. These were readers from all over the world who, just like me, felt homeless, and were those also seeking a safe haven where they could let down their heavy suitcases, unzip their heavy coats, and breathe.

It's these brave readers who gave me the light I needed to navigate many dark nights in solitude, and it is to them that I dedicate this book. Thank you, Lighters, for being there and walking beside me—Very Good Light is and will always be a love letter to you.

That being said, I could not have written this book if it weren't for the Pretty Boys who walked this earth before me. It was an honor to have researched each and every one of these individuals who paved a way for people like me to survive—and thrive!—in this world today. Thank you for being iconoclasts who pushed culture forward and made seismic shifts in the process. We've seen change in each decade from 50,000 BCE. We still have a ways to go, but I do hope that in another decade (or century), we'll look back and see the strides we as a civilization have made.

I am also thankful that I had this book to write during arguably the most difficult year of our lives—2020 with its pandemic and social uprisings. While I, too, was anxious and depressed, it was researching and writing this book that allowed me to escape the painful present and travel to different times and locations around the world. What a luxury it was to be able to time travel, meeting the most powerfully pretty people from years past. I am deeply indebted to all of these individuals.

I'm also thankful for the blessings from Higher Beings. Some might say the Universe, I say God. I believe in manifestation and I put it out there that I wanted to write this book back in 2017. Not knowing about the ins and outs of the publishing industry—from getting an agent to selling an idea for a book!—I asked the Powers that Be very detailed requests. Namely, that I needed someone to literally email me out of the blue, laying everything out, and helping me with every step of the way.

Almost exactly two years later to the date, an editor did just that. Her name is Jenny Xu and she informed me she worked for a publisher called Houghton Mifflin Harcourt. In her very thoughtful and friendly email, she expressed how much of a fan she was of Very Good Light, how she was reaching out to see if I had a book in me, and if I'd be interested in writing one. From that day forward, I realized that this book was given to me as a gift for a higher purpose. I was chosen as merely a vessel for the Universe to get this out there. Call me wuwu, but I still get goosebumps thinking about that day and am forever grateful. My life was forever changed.

Next came finding an agent. "Do you have one?" Jenny asked me one day over the phone. "Of course not!" I replied, being the amateur author I was. "You mean, someone would want to represent me?" I quickly got to work querying agents from recommendations. I finally landed upon not one, but *two* of the best agents in the business. They are Katherine Latshaw from Folio Literary, and Annie Hwang, from Ayesha Pande Literary. I owe both of you so much for not only believing in this book, but me as a first-time author. Thank you both for taking a chance on me. Your patience and your grace will never be forgotten. Skincare tips for life!

They say it takes a village to write a book. I'm thankful to many uncles and aunts who have pored over hundreds of hours to make this baby come to life. Thank you to Team HMH: Deb Brody for believing in this book, Mark Robinson and Christopher Moisan for your care on the art and conviction, and Christina Stambaugh, Marina Padakis Lowry, Ivy McFadden, Kevin Watt, Bridget Nocera, and Julie Yeater. This book only came alive through Paul Tuller's illustrations and Raphael Geroni for the beautiful cover and designing the pages.

Writing and researching this book for over a year (again, especially during a pandemic and quarantine) meant that I was stuck, enduring a lot of hours stuck in my home office. For the many late nights I thank LaCroix, Pringles, and double-shot Nespresso iced lattes. Oh, yes, and friends.

These include so many people who are closer to me than kin: Sarah Y., thank you so much for reading over every chapter and having thoughtful conversations with me. Huge shoutout to my LA family: Sarah Springer, Micah, Akemi, Patrick, Eddie Buck, Esther, Won, Jason, Bukunmi, Amber Kallor, Olivia, Mama Helen Koo, Marshall Bang, Chester Lockhart, Celeste Perez, Jenn King, Shelly Yo, Susan Cho, Karen Park, and Simone Oliver. My ARMY family: Connie Kuo, Brittany, and Janelle—thank you so much for always giving me space to air out my thoughts (and also for letting me use Jungkook and Jimin interchangeably, *borahae!*). And of course, to BTS Army for your support online and everywhere—I wrote this book thinking about you all and how to make you proud.

Huge thank you to Amerie for giving me words of wisdom—truly, you are a gem and I love you so much. Thank you for early endorsements, Joe Zee, Nicola Formichetti, and Charlotte Cho. My NYC fam: Charlotte (again) and Dave Cho (and Rambo!) and Baby Cho—THANK YOU for being my family away from home. ChoBNB forever! Joyce Lee, Liah Yoo, Jessica Shim, Dr. Claire, and Sydney. Oh, my momager, Susan Hong (and her new daughter, Lily!), Ann Yee, Adam Mansuroglu, Kenny, Jenni Lee, Jenny Lin, Bianca, Ian, Kristan, Sarah Spiegelman-Richter, and Slayrizz. Maki love you all.

Much gratitude for many of the interviews including Courtney Lazore, Professor Richard McBride, and Channing Joseph, among so many others.

My team at Very Good Light and Good Light beauty: Michael Engert, Leif Glynn, Lindsey Roberts, Alex and the Center Fam—you have all been so gracious and so accommodating and so patient to my unruly schedule. I appreciate you all! My (forever) interns: Isla and Olivia, thank you for encouraging me to the very end. My advisors: Georgie Greville, Joyce Kim, Arienne Thompson Plourde, Garrett Munce, and Z Reitano—you all are so special and I look up to each of you so much.

My Colorado family: Michelle, April, Gloria, Mavis, Erica, Pom and Vickie + all the Moons, Joanna, Danny + Kim Family, and Aaron. Also to Diane Nguyen and Victoria Kim—thank you for being my first supporters and my only friends from high school. My *gomo,* Young Mi, for your strength and resilience. My *samchon,* Joshua, for your grace and endurance.

My cousins: Andrew and Matthew Kim, Lisa Woods and Jacob Yi, LOVE YOU ALL—you all are my faves but don't tell anyone. Stacey, Eric, Juwon, and Jubin, love you guys.

Saving the most important for last: my biological family. Thank you to my mother and father, Sun Chin Yi and Sung Yong Yi, who had to endure my many ups and downs. Thank you for your patience, understanding, unconditional love—and for feeding me. I'm forever indebted to you both and hope you are proud of this book, after all, it's dedicated to you. To my grandmother Chong Chung Yo, who passed in March while I was writing this book: without seeing this book published, you were and still are my everything. Thank you for your wisdom, your beauty, your kindness, your love. Your emphasis on soft—from your voice, your velvety hands, your gaze—allowed me as a Korean man to be comfortable in my own skin.

My sister Jamie and brother-in-law Will, both of you deserve an award for being super-human-beings. For one, I love you guys and hope you make more children. Thank you for your unconditional love, allowing me to move into your then–South Carolina home, crashing your first year of marriage, and all of the fond memories that came from that time.

Finally, to the human being I cherish the most and who filled quarantine with joy and hope: Everett Jihu Choe. You are my first nephew and I wrote this book as a special gift to you. I hope this book will help you along your own journey into adulthood and will empower you to know that you are perfect just the way you are. And if ever you may forget, samchon is here to remind you of just how special—and powerful and wonderful and *magical*—you are. Now go change the world, we need you.

To all the pretty boys out there in the world: Cheers to us. We're here. We're loud. We've arrived and we aren't going anywhere.

May *good* light the way . . .

$\mathcal{N}$ OTES

ALL HISTORY IS INCONCLUSIVE TO SOME DEGREE. AFTER ALL, humans are subjective by nature. As such, this entire book is pieced together with a variety of sources in an attempt to create a clearer picture of reality and truth. Some are primary, while others are secondary. The notes below are what I've studied and it is my hope that they can help with anyone else searching for more clues to our vibrant pasts. May this road map illuminate your curiosities and lead your researching journeys.

Why Did Men Stop Wearing Makeup?

Joanna Bourke, "The Great Male Renunciation: Men's Dress Reform in Inter-War Britain," *Journal of Design History* 9, no. 1 (March 1996): 23–33.

Michael Zakim, *Ready-Made Democracy: A History of Men's Dress in the American Republic, 1760–1860* (Chicago: University of Chicago Press, 2003).

Nancy Tomes, *The Gospel of Germs: Men, Women, and the Microbe in American Life* (Cambridge, MA: Harvard University Press, 1999), 159.

Matt Houlbrook, "The Man with the Powder Puff in Interwar London," *Historical Journal* 50, no. 1 (March 2007): 145–171.

Thomas Lacquer, *Making Sex: Body and Gender from the Greeks to Freud* (Cambridge, MA: Harvard University Press, 1992).

Michael Kimmel, *Manhood in America, A Cultural History* (New York: Oxford University Press, 2011).

"TB's Surprising Results," PBS, https://www.pbs.org/wgbh/americanexperience/features/plague-know/.

Franklin Johnson, "The Masculine Woman," *Christian Repository & Home Circle,* September 1887.

Kathy Peiss, *Hope in a Jar: The Making of America's Beauty Culture* (Philadelphia: University of Pennsylvania Press, 2011).

Sarah Gold McBride, "Power Is on the Side of the Beard," U.S. History Scene, https://ushistoryscene.com/article/beards/.

Sara Damiano, "The Decline of Barbers? Or, the Risks and Rewards of Quantitative Analysis," *The Junto* (blog), July 23, 2014, https://earlyamericanists.com/2014/07/23/guest-post-the-decline-of-barbers-or-the-risks-and-rewards-of-quantitative-analysis/.

Bob Batchelor, *The 1900s* (Westport, CT: Greenwood Press, 2002), 99.

Tangee Natural Lipstick, *Vogue,* August, 1943.

Neanderthal (50,000 BCE)

Christopher Joyce, "Study: Neanderthals Wore Jewelry and Makeup," NPR, January 12, 2010, https://www.npr.org/templates/story/story.php?storyId=122466430.

Alok Jha, "Neanderthals May Have Been First Human Species to Create Cave Paintings," *The Guardian,* June 14, 2012, https://www.theguardian.com/science/2012/jun/14/neanderthals-first-create-cave-paintings.

João Zilhão, email interview by David Yi, January 9, 2020.

Ramses the Great

John Toedt, Darrell Koza, and Kathleen Van Cleef-Toedt, *Chemical Composition of Everyday Products* (Westport, CT: Greenwood Publishing Group, 2005), 4.

Michael Bernstein, "Ancient Egyptian Cosmetics: 'Magical' Makeup May Have Been Medicine for Eye Disease," American Chemical Society, January 11, 2010, https://www.acs.org/content/acs/en/pressroom/newsreleases/2010/january/ancient-egyptian-cosmetics.html.

Rebecca Kreston, "Ophthalmology of the Pharaohs: Antimicrobial Kohl Eyeliner in Ancient Egypt," *Discover,* August 20, 2012, https://www.discovermagazine.com/health/ophthalmology-of-the-pharaohs-antimicrobial-kohl-eyeliner-in-ancient-egypt.

Hatshepsut

Joshua J. Mark, "Hatshepsut," *Ancient History Encyclopedia,* October 19, 2016, https://www.ancient.eu/hatshepsut/.

Victoria Sherrow, *Encyclopedia of Hair: A Cultural History* Westport, CT: Greenwood Press, 2006), 127.

Victoria Sherrow, *For Appearances' Sake: The Historical Encyclopedia of Good Looks, Beauty, and Grooming* (Phoenix, AZ: Oryx Press, 2001), 113.

Bob Brier and A. Hoyt Hobbs, *Daily Life of the Ancient Egyptians* (Westport, CT : Greenwood Publishing Group, 2008), 21.

Elizabeth B. Wilson, "The Queen Who Would Be King," *Smithsonian Magazine,* September 2006.

Cyrus the Great

Pierre Briant, *From Cyrus to Alexander: A History of the Persian Empire* (University Park, PA: Eisenbrauns, 2002), 226.

Firouzeh Mirrazavi, "Perfume and Perfume Manufacturing in Ancient Iran," Iran Review, March 25, 2013, http://www.iranreview.org/content/Documents/Perfume_Perfume_Manufacturing_in_Iran.htm.

Xenophon, *Cyropaedia,* vol. 2 (Portsmouth, NH: W. Heinemann, 1914), 325.

Lloyd Llewellyn-Jones, *King and Court in Ancient Persia 559 to 331 BCE* (Edinburgh: Edinburgh University Press, 2014).

Alexander the Great

Ravi K. Puri and Raman Puri, *Natural Aphrodisiacs: Myth or Reality* (self-pub., Xlibris US, 2011), 149.

Jennifer Peace Rhind, *Fragrance and Wellbeing: Plant Aromatics and Their Influence on the Psyche* (London: Singing Dragon, 2013), 81

Elena Vosnaki, "Ancient Fragrant Lore: The Time of Alexander (Part 4)," Fragrantica, https://www.fragrantica.com/news/Ancient-Fragrant-Lore-The-Time-of-Alexander-Part-4—5933.html.

Xenophon, *Cyropaedia,* vol. 2 (Portsmouth, NH: W. Heinemann, 1914), 325.

Hwarang

Edward Shultz and Hugh H. W. Kang, *The Koguryo Annals of the Samguk Sagi* (Gyeonggi-do, South Korea: The Academy of Korean Studies Press, 2012), 131.

Scott Shaw, *Hapkido: Korean Art of Self-Defense* (Clarendon, VT: Tuttle Publishing, 1997).

"신라시대의 화장," *Naver,* blog post, https://terms.naver.com/entry.nhn?docId=776028&mobile&cid=42939&categoryId=42939.

Wanne J. Joe, *A Cultural History of Modern Korea: A History of Korean Civilization* (Seoul: Hollym International Corp., 2000).

Courtney Lazore, "The Hwarang Warriors: Silla's Flower Boys," *Dartmouth Quarterly of East Asian Studies,* Fall 2014.

Richard D. McBride, "Silla Buddhism and the 'Hwarang segi' Manuscripts," *Korean Studies* 31 (2007): 19–38.

Kim Chongguk, Kim Chinman, David Chung, and Richard Rutt, *Transactions of the Korea Brand of the Royal Asiatic Society, Volume XXXVII* (Seoul, South Korea:Royal Asiatic Society Korea Branch, 1961).

Aleksandra Jachimowicz, Ashley Kim, Siran Wang, Yu Xia, and He Zhang, "The Influence of Chang-An Culture to Korea and Japan: Clothing," Stony Brook University research project, https://you.stonybrook.edu/changanculture/clothing/.

Kim Myong Hee, "유신랑의 화장법," *BNT News,* August 6, 2009, https://bnt-news.hankyung.com/apps/news.view?aid=200908062217293&media=bnt MobileLife.

Richard McBride, phone interview by David Yi, March 9, 2019.

Vikings

Rym Ghazal, "When the Arabs Met the Vikings: New Discovery Suggests Ancient Links," *The National,* May 6, 2015, https://www.thenational.ae/world/when-the-arabs-met-the-vikings-new-discovery-suggests-ancient-links-1.125718.

Anita Croy, *Baffling Bathing Customs* (New York: Gareth Stevens Publishing, 2018), 13.

Steven P. Ashby, *A Viking Way of Life* (Stroud, UK: Amberley Publishing Limited, 2014).

Octavia Randolph, "Your Legal Rights Under Alfred, King of Wessex," Octavia.net, https://octavia.net/your-legal-rights-under-aelfred-king-of-wessex.

Carolyn Emerick, "Vikings: The Pretty Boys of the Middle Ages?," *Celtic Guide* 2, no. 8 (2013), https://www.medievalists.net/wp-content/uploads/2013/07/Viking-Article-Carolyn-Emerick.pdf.

Thomas DuBois, *Nordic Religions in the Viking Age* (Philadelphia: University of Pennsylvania Press, 1999).

King Louis XIV

Kimberly Chrisman-Campbell, "The King of Couture," *The Atlantic,* September 1, 2015.

Lucas Reilly, "Why Did People Wear Powdered Wigs," *Mental Floss,* June 29, 2012.

Peter Burke, *The Fabrication of Louis XIV* (Yale University Press, 1994).

Michael Kwass, "Big Hair: A Wig History of Consumption in Eighteenth-Century France," History Cooperative, https://historycooperative.org/journal/big-hair-a-wig-history-of-consumption-in-eighteenth-century-france/.

Joan DeJean, *The Essence of Style: How the French Invented High Fashion, Fine Food, Chic Cafes, Style, Sophistication, and Glamour* (New York: Simon and Schuster, 2007).

Victoria Sherrow, *Encyclopedia of Hair: A Cultural History* (Westport, CT: Greenwood, 2006).

John Woodfored, *The Strange Story of False Hair* (Drake Publishers, 1972).

Macaroni

Joseph Twadell Shipley, *The Origins of English Words* (Baltimore: Johns Hopkins University Press, 2001).

Peter McNeil, *Pretty Gentlemen* (New Haven, CT: Yale University Press, 2018).

Amelia Rauser, "Hair, Authenticity, and the Self-Made Macaroni," *Eighteenth-Century Studies* 38, no. 1 (Fall 2004): 101–7.

"Julius Soubise," *100 Great Black Britons* (blog), https://100greatblackbritons.com/bios/julius_soubise.html.

Monica L. Miller, *Slave to Fashion: Black Dandyism and the Styling of Black Diasporic Identity* (Durham, NC: Duke University Press, 2009).

Hunter Oatman-Stanford, "That Time the French Aristocracy Was Obsessed with Sexy Face Stickers," *Collectors Weekly,* May 4, 2017, https://www.collectorsweekly.com/articles/sexy-face-stickers/

Cleaning Up

C. Bushdid, M. O. Magnasco, L. B. Vosshall, and A. Keller, "Humans Can Discriminate More Than 1 Trillion Olfactory Stimuli," *Science,* March 21, 2014.

Katherine Ashenburg, *The Dirt on Clean: An Unsanitized History* (New York: Farrar, Straus and Giroux, 2014).

Amanda Foreman, "The Long Road to Cleanliness," *Wall Street Journal,* October 4, 2019.

Upinder Singh, *A History of Ancient and Early Medieval India: From the Stone Age to the 12th Century* (Delhi, India: Pearson Education India, 2008).

Vogue, Conde Nast Publications, July 1974.

Ian Rotherham, *Spas and Spa Visiting* (New York: Bloomsbury Publishing, 2014), 11.

Insight Guides, *Insight Guides South Korea* (Washington, DC: APA, 2016).

Coming Clean with Beauty

"Little-Known or Unknown Facts Regarding Elizabeth I's Death," Royal Museums Greenwich blog, https://www.rmg.co.uk/discover/explore/little-known-or-unknown-facts-regarding-queen-elizabeth-is-death.

Beau Brummell

Ian Kelly, *Beau Brummell: The Ultimate Man of Style* (New York: Simon and Schuster, 2013).

Modern Sanitation: Vol. 2 (Louisville, KY: Standard Sanitary Mfg, 1906), 19.

Black Panther Party

Ayana Byrd and Lori Tharps, *Hair Story: Untangling the Roots of Black Hair in America* (New York: St. Martin's Press, 2002).

Steven Thrasher, "A Personal and Political History of the Afro," BuzzFeed, November 5, 2013, https://www.buzzfeednews.com/article/steventhrasher/a-personal-and-political-history-of-the-afro.

Huey P. Newton, *Revolutionary Suicide* (New York: Penguin, 2009).

Kathleen Cleaver: Interview on Natural Hair, Interview (Education Video Group, 1968): https://www.youtube.com/watch?v=JUna84ztulU.

(Pretty) Boys to Men

Bruce Beehler, "Plumes of Paradise," National Wildlife Federation, February 1, 2003, https://www.nwf.org/en/Magazines/National-Wildlife/2003/Plumes-of-Paradise.

Lindsay Brown, Jean-Bernard Carillet, and Anna Kaminski, *Lonely Planet Papua New Guinea & Solomon Islands* (New York: Lonely Planet Global Limited, 2016).

Erin Kenny and Elizabeth Gackstetter Nichols, *Beauty Around the World: A Cultural Encyclopedia* (Goleta, CA: ABC-CLIO, 2017), 318.

Victoria R. Williams, *Indigenous Peoples: An Encyclopedia of Culture, History, and Threats to Survival* (Goleta, CA : ABC-CLIO, 2020), 568.

Dr. Kate Lister, "Sex in Our Strange World," *Vice,* December 12, 2019, https://amuse.vice.com/en_us/article/neg5g8/wodaabe-wife-stealing-sex.

K'inich Janaab' Pakal

"The Maya Concept of Beauty," History on the Net, July 29, 2020, https://www.historyonthenet.com/the-maya-concept-of-beauty.

Norman Hammond, "The Maya Suffered for Their Looks," *The Times* (London), January 13, 2009, http://www.latinamericanstudies.org/maya/maya-looks.htm.

Mary Miller, "Extreme Makeover," *Archaeology* 62, no. 1 (January/February 2009), https://archive.archaeology.org/0901/abstracts/maya.html.

"Ancient Maya Endured Unspeakable Pain to Make Themselves Beautiful," The Free Library, https://www.thefreelibrary.com/Ancient+Maya+endured+unspeakable+pain+to+make+themselves+beautiful-a0212309995.

Beyond the Binary

Jessica Hinchy, *Governing Gender and Sexuality in Colonial India: The Hijra* (Cambridge, UK: Cambridge University Press, 2020).

Stephen O. Murray, *Homosexualites* (Chicago: University of Chicago Press, 2000), 291.

Jeannette Marie Mageo, *Theorizing Self in Samoa* (Ann Arbor, MI: University of Michigan Press, 1998), 291.

Richard Totman, *The Third Sex: Kathoey—Thailand's Ladyboys* (London: Souvenir Press, 2004).

Let's Get It Clear

Loren Zech, Bryce Turner, and Scott A. Norton, "Presidential Practice of Dermatology," *JAMA Dermatology* 149, no. 9 (September 2013): 1032.

John Hambling and Philip Hopkins, *Psychosomatic Disorders in Adolescents and Young Adults: Proceedings of a Conference Held by the Society for Psychosomatic Research at the Royal College of Physicians, London November 1960* (New York: Elsevier, 2013).

Janet. H. Moore, "The Nightingale Facial," *Wall Street Journal,* December 14, 2001, https://www.wsj.com/articles/SB1008292800778950720.

Gabrielle Hatfield, *Encyclopedia of Folk Medicine: Old World and New World Traditions* (Goleta, CA: ABC-CLIO, 2004).

Humyra Tabasum, Tanzeel Ahmad, Farzana Anjum, and Hina Rehman, "The Historical Panorama of Acne Vulgaris," *Journal of Pakistan Association of Dermatologists* 23, no. 3 (2013): 315–19, https://applications.emro.who.int/imemrf/J_Pak_Assoc_Dermatol/J_Pak_Assoc_Dermatol_2013_23_3_315_319.pdf.

Ruqiya Shama Tareen et al., *Pediatric Psychodermatology: A Clinical Manual of Child and Adolescent Psychocutaneous Disorders* (Boston: Walter de Gruyter, 2012).

Gerd Plewig and Albert M. Kligman, "History of Acne and Rosacea," in *Acne and Rosacea* (Berlin/Heidelberg: Springer, 2000).

Susruthi Rajanala and Neelam A. Vashi, "Cleopatra and Sour Milk—The Ancient Practice of Chemical Peeling," *JAMA Dermatology* 153, no. 10 (October 2017): 1006, https://jamanetwork.com/journals/jamadermatology/article-abstract/2657249.

Graeme Donald, *The Mysteries of History: Unravelling the Truth from the Myths of Our Past* (London: Michael O'Mara Books, 2018).

Max Factor

"The Max Factor Story," Max Factor, https://www.maxfactor.com/en-ae/our-brand/max-factor-story.

John Updike, "Makeup and Make Believe," *New Yorker,* August 25, 2008, https://www.newyorker.com/magazine/2008/09/01/makeup-and-make-believe.

Cecilia Rasmussen, "A Man Who Changed the Faces of Hollywood," *Los Angeles Times,* March 21, 1999, https://www.latimes.com/archives/la-xpm-1999-mar-21-me-19559-story.html.

Maisie Skidmore, "How Max Factor Invented Modern Makeup," *AnOther,* August 30, 2016, https://www.anothermag.com/fashion-beauty/9005/how-max-factor-invented-modern-makeup.

John Updike, *Higher Gossip: Essays and Criticism* (New York: Random House, 2011).

Stella Rose Saint Clair, "Makeup Masters: The History of Max Factor," Beautylish, February 12, 2014, https://www.beautylish.com/a/vxspr/the-history-of-max-factor.

Black Beauty Brands Broke Barriers

Shammara Lawrence, "Carol's Daughter Founder Lisa Price Reflects on the Iconic Hair-Care Brand's 25-Year Run," *Allure,* May 30, 2018, https://www.allure.com/story/carols-daughter-lisa-price-interview-25-year-anniversary.

Christopher Robert Reed, *The Rise of Chicago's Black Metropolis, 1920–1929* (Champaign, IL:University of Illinois Press, 2011).

Madam C. J. Walker, *Text Book of the Madam C.J. Walker Schools of Beauty Culture* (Indianapolis: Manufacturing Company, American, 1940).

Colleen Cottet, "Love for Sale: The Graphic Art of Valmor Products," *Chicago Reader,* https://www.chicagoreader.com/chicago/love-for-sale-the-graphic-art-of-valmor-products/Event?oid=18560640.

Victoria Sherrow, *Encyclopedia of Hair: A Cultural History* (Westport, CT: Greenwood Press, 2006), 197.

Jean E. Snyder, *Harry T. Burleigh: From the Spiritual to the Harlem Renaissance* (Champaign, IL: University of Illinois Press, 2016), 141.

"Black Is Beautiful: The Emergence of Black Culture and Identity in the 60s and 70s," Smithsonian National Museum of African American History & Culture, https://nmaahc.si.edu/blog-post/black-beautiful-emergence-black-culture-and-identity-60s-and-70s.

Jillian Steinhauer, "Uncovering the Soul of the 'Black Is Beautiful' Movement," *New York Times,* July 3, 2019, https://www.nytimes.com/2019/07/03/arts/design/kwame-brathwaite-black-is-beautiful-photography.html.

Susannah Walker, *Style and Status: Selling Beauty to African American Women, 1920–1975* (Lexington, KY: University Press of Kentucky, 2007), 171.

Robin Givhan, "What Happened to Fashion Fair?" *Washington Post,* October 27, 2015, https://www.washingtonpost.com/lifestyle/style/what-happened-to-fashion-fair-why-the-black-cosmetics-brand-is-so-hard-to-find/2015/10/27/17416cf0-72be-11e5-8d93-0af317ed58c9_story.html.

Kristin Larson, "Can Fashion Fair Cosmetics Make a Comeback?" *Fortune,* September 17, 2019, https://fortune.com/2019/09/17/can-fashion-fair-cosmetics-make-a-comeback/.

Nadia Mustafa, "Women in Fashion," *Time,* February 9, 2004, http://content.time.com/time/specials/packages/article/0,28804,2015519_2015510_2015477,00.html

Rudolph Valentino

Thomas Mallon, "Those Lips, Those Eyes," *New Yorker,* May 12, 2003, https://www.newyorker.com/magazine/2003/05/19/those-lips-those-eyes.

Gilbert King, "The 'Latin Lover' and His Enemies," *Smithsonian,* June 13, 2012, https://www.smithsonianmag.com/history/the-latin-lover-and-his-enemies-119968944/

Ulrike Blume-Peytavi, David A. Whiting, and Ralph M. Trueb, *Hair Growth and Disorders* (New York: Springer Science & Business Media), 534.

"Valentino Seeking Fight with Editor," *New York Times,* July 21, 1926, https://timesmachine.nytimes.com/timesmachine/1926/07/21/98493376.pdf.

Clark Gable

Chrystopher J. Spicer, *Clark Gable: Biography, Filmography, Bibliography* (Jefferson, NC: McFarland, Incorporated, Publishers, 2002).

Warren G. Harris, *Clark Gable: A Biography* (New York: Crown, 2010), 109.

David Bret, *Clark Gable: Tormented Star* (New York: Aurum Press, 2014).

John Farr, "Clark Gable: King of Hollywood," *HuffPost,* May 1, 2013, https://www.huffpost.com/entry/clark-gable-king-of-holly_b_1244759.

Shi Pei Pu

Joyce Wadler, "Shi Pei Pu, Singer, Spy and 'M. Butterfly,' Dies at 70," *New York Times,* July 1, 2009, https://www.nytimes.com/2009/07/02/world/asia/02shi.html.

Joyce Wadler, "The True Story of M. Butterfly; The Spy Who Fell in Love with a Shadow," *New York Times,* August 15, 1993.

Pat Launer, "M. Butterfly at the North Coast Repertory Theatre," *KPBS,* August 25, 1993, https://patlauner.com/review/m-butterfly-at-the-north-coast-repertory-theatre/.

Karina Eileraas, *Between Image and Identity* (Lanham, MD: Lexington Books, 2007), 31.

RuPaul

Kristen Chuba and Allison Crist, "Emmys: RuPaul Wins Best Reality Host 4th Year in a Row, Typing Jeff Probst's Record," *Hollywood Reporter,* September 14, 2019, https://www.hollywoodreporter.com/news/rupauls-drag-race-wins-emmy-best-reality-host-4th-time-1238652.

Mac McClelland, "RuPaul: The King of Queens," *Rolling Stone,* October 4, 2013, https://www.rollingstone.com/movies/movie-news/rupaul-the-king-of-queens-184143/.

Richard Lawson, "RuPaul: The Philosopher Queen," *Vanity Fair,* November 20, 2019, https://www.vanityfair.com/hollywood/2019/11/rupaul-cover-story.

Drag Queens: A Herstory

Bernadette Deron, "The Evolution of the Art of Drag in 33 Stunning, Historical Images," All That's Interesting, December 15, 2018, https://allthatsinteresting.com/history-of-drag-queens.

Channing Gerard Joseph, "The First Drag Queen Was a Former Slave," *The Nation,* February 17, 2020, https://www.thenation.com/article/society/drag-queen-slave-ball/.

Regan Shrumm, "Who Takes the Cake? The History of the Cakewalk," National Museum of American History, May 18, 2016, https://americanhistory.si.edu/blog/who-takes-cake-history-cakewalk.

John S. Farmer and William Ernest Henley, *Slang and Its Analogues Past and Present: A Dictionary, Historical and Comparative, of the Heterodox Speech of All Classes of Society for More Than Three Hundred Years,* vol. 2 (London: Harrison and Sons, December 21, 1891).

Oliver Stabbe, "Queens and Queers: The Rise of Drag Ball Culture in the 1920s," *O Say Can You See?* (blog), National Museum of American History, April 11, 2016, https://americanhistory.si.edu/blog/queens-and-queers-rise-drag-ball-culture-1920s.

"Hamilton Lodge Ball Is Scene of Splendor," *New York Age,* February 22, 1930, via https://www.queermusicheritage.com/nov2014hamilton.html.

"Arresting Dress: A Timeline of Anti-Cross-Dressing Laws in the United States," *PBS Newshour Weekend,* May 31, 2015, https://www.pbs.org/newshour/nation/arresting-dress-timeline-anti-cross-dressing-laws-u-s.

Billy Porter

Vincent Boucher and Ingridt Schmidt, "Tonys: Billy Porter's Pro-Choice Look Features Uterus Motif," *Hollywood Reporter,* June 9, 2019, https://www.hollywoodreporter.com/news/billy-porter-2019-tony-awards-look-has-pro-choice-uterus-motif-1216756.

Billy Porter, "Oh My, How Things Have Changed . . . ," blog post, https://billyporter.com/blog/2017/1/15/oh-my-how-things-have-changed.

Billy Porter, "The First Time I Refused to Keep Playing a Stereotype," *New York Times,* November 21, 2017, https://www.nytimes.com/2017/11/21/theater/billy-porter-the-first-time-i-refused-to-keep-playing-a-stereotype.html.

Frank Ocean's Blond(e) Moment

Diane Solway, "Frank Ocean Makes Moves Like Nobody Else," *W Magazine,* September 30, 2019, https://www.wmagazine.com/story/frank-ocean-cover-story-interview/.

Emmett Cruddas and Vegyn, "Frank Ocean Is Peerless," *GQ,* January 10, 2019, https://www.gq.com/story/frank-ocean-is-peerless.

Tom Jackson, "Frank Ocean," *Gayletter,* April 2019.

Jason King and Ann Powers, "Detangling Frank Ocean's 'Blonde': What It Is and Isn't," The Record (NPR), August 22, 2016, https://www.npr.org/sections/therecord/2016/08/22/490918270/detangling-frank-oceans-blonde-what-it-is-and-isnt.

Sam Wolfson, "Frank Ocean's Blonde Dissected: 'A Cultural Artefact That Deserves to Be Studied,'" *The Guardian,* May 21, 2018, https://www.theguardian.com/music/2018/may/21/frank-ocean-album-blonde-dissect-cole-cuchna.

Bad Bunny

Albert Serna Jr., "Gay, Latino and Macho," *Substance,* September 10, 2014, https://substance.media/gay-latino-and-macho-c931e022ec47.

Jhoni Jackson, "Bad Bunny Just Hits Different," *Paper,* June 6, 2019, https://www.papermag.com/bad-bunny-2638705133.html?rebelltitem=1#rebelltitem1.

Gabriela Berlingeri, "Bad Bunny in Captivity," *Rolling Stone,* May 14, 2020, https://www.rollingstone.com/music/music-features/bad-bunny-cover-story-lockdown-puerto-rico-new-albums-996871/.

You've Got Nail

"Belles of Old Babylon Were Manicured Men," *St. Petersburg Times,* March 1, 1950.

Natasha Sheldon, "Looks That Kill: 11 Impossible Beauty Standards from History," History Collection, https://historycollection.com/changing-face-fashion-11-historical-standards-beauty/5/.

James Robinson, "Fatimid Flask Reliquary," *Treasures of Heaven* exhibition, Cleveland Museum of Art with the British Museum, https://projects.mcah.columbia.edu/treasuresof heaven/relics/Fatimid-Flask-Reliquary.php.

JR Thorpe, "7 Bizarre Beliefs About Nails From History," *Bustle,* August 9, 2016, https://www.bustle.com/articles/176933-7-bizarre-beliefs-about-nails-from-history.

Ji Baek, *Rescue Your Nails* (New York: Workman Publishing, 2015), 4.

Gabriella Baki and Kenneth S. Alexander, *Introduction to Cosmetic Formulation and Technology* (Hoboken, NJ: Wiley, 2015), 420.

Lord Byron

John Cordy Jeaffreson, *The Real Lord Byron: New Views of the Poet's Life* (London: Hurst & Blackett), 93.

Louise Foxcroft, "Lord Byron: The Celebrity Diet Icon," BBC, January 3, 2012, https://www.bbc.com/news/magazine-16351761.

Don Carlos Seitz, *Artemus Ward (Charles Farrar Browne): A Biography and Bibliography* (New York: Harper, 1919), 161.

Megan Gressor and Kerry Cook, *An Affair to Remember: The Greatest Love Stories of All Time* (Beverly, MA: Fair Winds Press, 2004), 101

The Lugubrious Tales of Body Modifications Past

B. O. Rogers, "A Chronologic History of Cosmetic Surgery," *Bulletin of the New York Academy of Medicine* 47, no. 3 (March 1971): 265–302, https://www.ncbi.nlm.nih.gov/pmc/articles/PMC1749866/?page=1.

"Pictures of First Person to Undergo Plastic Surgery Released," *Telegraph* (UK), August 28, 2008, https://www.telegraph.co.uk/news/uknews/2636507/Pictures-of-first-person-to-undergo-plastic-surgery-released.html.

Arjan Das, "Sushruta, the First Surgeon," *Telegraph of India,* September 23, 2018, https://www.telegraphindia.com/opinion/the-first-surgeon/cid/1669902.

Marija D Pecanac, "Development of Plastic Surgery," *Medicinski Pregled* 68, no. 5–6 (May–June 2015): 199–204, https://pubmed.ncbi.nlm.nih.gov/26234029/.

Little Richard

Robert Chalmers, "Legend: Little Richard," *GQ,* March 29, 2012, https://www.gq-magazine.co.uk/article/gq-men-of-the-year-2010-little-richard-legend.

John Waters, "When John Waters Met Little Richard," *The Guardian,* November 27, 2010, https://www.theguardian.com/music/2010/nov/28/john-waters-met-little-richard.

Kevin Naulls, "What I Wish My Parents Had Said When I Came Out as Gay," CBC, October 11, 2019, https://www.cbc.ca/parents/learning/view/what-i-wish-my-parents-had-said-when-i-came-out-as-gay.

Richard Corliss, "Tutti Frutti," *Time,* October 21, 2011, https://entertainment.time.com/2011/10/24/the-all-time-100-songs/slide/tutti-frutti-little-richard/.

Marc Myers, "Richard, the First," *Wall Street Journal,* August 10, 2010, https://www.wsj.com/articles/SB10001424052748703545604575407661245246210.

Parke Puterbaugh, "Little Richard: 'I Am the Architect of Rock & Roll,'" *Rolling Stone,* April 19, 1990, https://www.rollingstone.com/music/music-features/little-richard-i-am-the-architect-of-rock-roll-121006/.

Associated Press, "David Bowie, Unpredictable Rock Superstar, Dead at 69," *Epoch Times,* January 11, 2016, https://www.theepochtimes.com/david-bowie-unpredictable-rock-superstar-dead-at-69_1938387.html.

Glam Rock

Jim Farber, "Growing Up Gay to a Glam Rock Soundtrack," *New York Times,* November 3, 2016, https://www.nytimes.com/2016/11/04/fashion/mens-style/growing-up-gay-glam-rock-queen-bowie-freddie-mercury.html.

Katie Rogers, "Was He Gay, Bisexual or Bowie? Yes," *New York Times,* January 13, 2016, https://www.nytimes.com/2016/01/14/style/was-he-gay-bisexual-or-bowie-yes.html.

David Bowie, "Doesn't It Look Like I'm Having Fun?" *The Guardian,* April 2, 2001, https://www.theguardian.com/culture/2001/apr/02/artsfeatures.davidbowie.

Simon Reynolds, *Shock and Awe* (New York: HarperCollins, 2016).

Jan Iles, "Whatever Happened to the Teenage Dream?" *Record and Popswop Mirror,* February 1, 1975, https://www.tilldawn.net/InterviewReviewStory/popswap.html.

Visual Kei

Loudwire, "X Japan's Yoshiki Talks Visual Kei Movement," YouTube video, 5:28, October 6, 2014, https://www.youtube.com/watch?v=cTJVVFGfCQI.

Annette Lynch and Mitchell D. Strauss, *Ethnic Dress in the United States: A Cultural Encyclopedia* (Lanham, MD: Rowman & Littlefield Publishers, 2014), 159.

Gavin Wright, Hugh T. Patrick, and Robert M. Stern, eds., *The Japanese Economy in Retrospect: Selected Papers by Gary R. Saxonhouse* (Singapore: World Scientific Publishing Company), 268.

Nick Chen, "Sects, Suicide & Speed Metal: The Unreal Story of X Japan," *Dazed Digital,* March 1, 2017, https://www.dazeddigital.com/music/article/34948/1/x-japan-we-are-x-speed-metal-band-david-lynch.

Lucy Dayman, "How Glam Rock Band X Japan Spearheaded the Nation's Most Unique Fashion Movement," *Culture Trip,* June 28, 2018, https://theculturetrip.com/asia/japan/articles/how-glam-rock-band-x-japan-spearheaded-the-nations-most-unique-fashion-movement/.

Boy George

Don Giller, "Boy George on Letterman, June 29, 1983," YouTube video, 11:06, June 22, 2016, https://www.youtube.com/watch?v=ePHwbiNqhBE.

Jeff Houck, "Donahue—Boy George and Culture Club (1984)," YouTube video, 46:50, Oct 16, 2017, https://www.youtube.com/watch?v=fLuypKBxFt0.

Laura Branigan Forever, "Boy George First time with Johnny Carson 1984," YouTube video, 12:15, August 27, 2013, https://www.youtube.com/watch?v=gsht3jLkMxo&t=651s.

Richard Harrington, "Boy George Rocks Bizarre," *Washington Post,* March 6, 1983, https://www.washingtonpost.com/archive/lifestyle/style/1983/03/06/boy-george-rocks-bizarre/6318194f-5cb5-4efb-a64a-15e4d11f924e/.

"The Ultimate Guide to the 1980s New Romantic Trend," Beyond Retro Vintage Clothing, blog post, September 6, 2018, https://www.beyondretro.com/blogs/news/the-ultimate-guide-to-the-1980s-new-romantic-trend.

Stan Hawkins, *Queerness in Pop Music: Aesthetics, Gender Norms, and Temporality* (New York: Routledge, 2015).

Ted Mico, "The Boy Bounces Back," *SPIN,* June 1989.

Karen DeYoung, "Boy George Located in Drug Case," *Washington Post,* July 10, 1986.

Steve Craig, *Men, Masculinity and the Media* (Newbury Park, CA: SAGE Publications, 1992), 54.

Club Kids

William Van Meter, "What Michael Alig's Club Kids Are Doing Now," *New York,* May 20, 2014, https://nymag.com/intelligencer/2014/05/what-michael-aligs-club-kids-are-doing-now.html.

Walt Cassidy, *New York: Club Kids: By Waltpaper* (Bologna, Italy: Damiani, 2019).

Sheila Flynn, "Where New York's Club Kids 80's and 90's are now," *Daily Mail,* September 4, 2017.

Harry Styles

Eliza Thompson, "Harry Styles's AMAs Suit Looks Like Everybody's Bedspread," *Cosmopolitan,* November 23, 2015.

"AMAs: What Was Harry Styles Thinking? 1D Star Shows Off Questionable Wardrobe Choice," *Stuff,* November 23, 2015, https://www.stuff.co.nz/entertainment/celebrities/74318662/amas-what-was-harry-styles-thinking-1d-star-shows-off-questionable-wardrobe-choice.

Rob Sheffield, "The Eternal Sunshine of Harry Styles," August 26, 2019, *Rolling Stone,* https://www.rolling-stone.com/music/music-features/harry-styles-cover-interview-album-871568/.

Cameron Crowe, "Harry Styles' New Direction," April 18, 2017, *Rolling Stone,* https://www.rollingstone.com/music/music-features/harry-styles-new-direction-119432/.

Troye Sivan

Eugenie Kelly, "Bazaar Man Troye Sivan on Clothes, Coming Out and His Hollywood Home Life," *Harper's Bazaar Australia,* September 28, 2019, https://www.harpersbazaar.com.au/celebrity/troye-sivan-bazaar-man-19346.

Michael Schulman, "Troye Sivan's Coming of Age," *New Yorker,* June 17, 2019, https://www.newyorker.com/magazine/2019/06/24/troye-sivans-coming-of-age.

BTS

Raisa Bruner, "How BTS Is Taking Over the World," *Time,* October 10, 2018, https://time.com/collection-post/5414052/bts-next-generation-leaders/.

Tamar Herman, "How BTS Took Over the World: A Timeline of the Group's Biggest Career Moments," *Billboard,* May 14, 2018, https://www.billboard.com/articles/columns/k-town/8455612/bts-takeover-timeline-bbmas.

Aja Romano, "BTS, the Band That Changed K-Pop, Explained," Vox, February 21, 2020, https://www.vox.com/culture/2018/6/13/17426350/bts-history-members-explained.

K-pop

JTBC Voyage, "Tapgol GD Yang Joon-Il's Rebecca," YouTube video, 13:30, December 11, 2019, https://www.youtube.com/watch?v=ePHwbiNqhBE.

"Amount of Money Spent on Cosmetics Purchase in South Korea from 2014-2016," Statista, https://www.statista.com/statistics/712561/south-korea-spending-on-cosmetics/.

Jessica Rapp, "South Korean Men Lead the World's Male Beauty Market. Will the West Ever Follow Suit?" CNN Style, March 3, 2020, https://www.cnn.com/style/article/south-korea-male-beauty-market-chanel/index.html.

INDEX

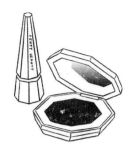

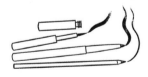

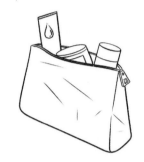

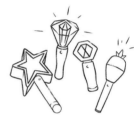